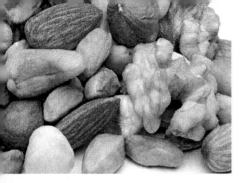
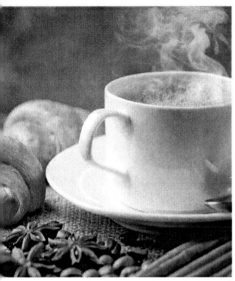
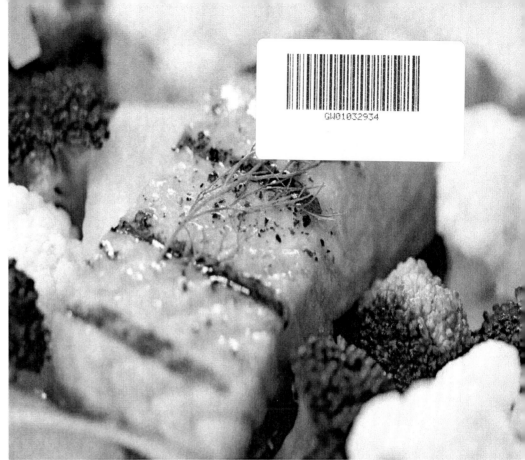

Acid Reflux Diet Cookbook
Companion Food Journal

60-day, detailed recording log to identify problem foods, drinks, meds, and habits.

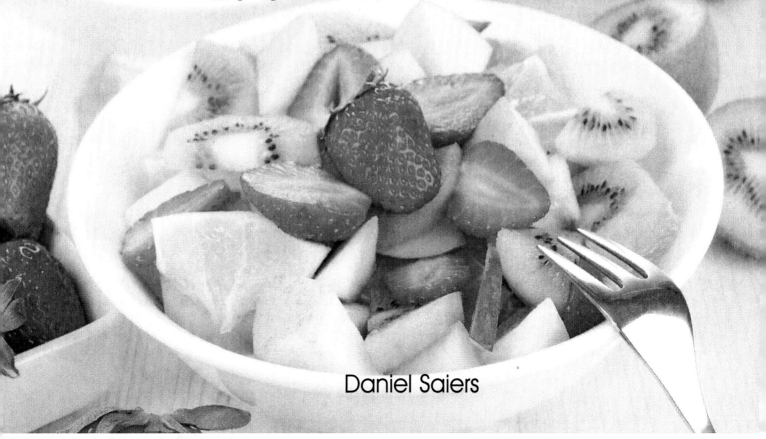

Daniel Saiers

Breakfast   Time: 8.15

List the foods you ate for breakfast.

Cornflakes with
milk.

Drink Cup of tea + milk.
○ room-temp ⊘ hot ○ cold

Drink Cup of tea + milk
○ room-temp ⊘ hot ○ cold

Physical symptoms after meal: ⊘ low ○ intense ○ non-existent
○ Belching   ⊘ Upper abdominal pain and discomfort
⊘ Nausea   ○ Difficulty or pain with swallowing
○ Stomach fullness or bloating   ○ Wheezing or dry cough

Other symptoms: Burning sensation, Hot + cold
spews
Post-breakfast energy level: ○ low ⊘ medium ○ high

Lunch   Time: 12.00

List the foods you ate for lunch.

2 slices wht Bread   Bag of L/Fat Crisps.
with honey Roast Ham
1 Lowfat yogurt

Drink Cup Tea + milk.
○ room-temp ⊘ hot ○ cold

Drink Glass of water
○ room-temp ○ hot ⊘ cold

Physical symptoms after meal: ○ low ⊘ intense ○ non-existent
○ Belching   ⊘ Upper abdominal pain and discomfort
⊘ Nausea   ○ Difficulty or pain with swallowing
⊘ Stomach fullness or bloating   ○ Wheezing or dry cough

Other symptoms: Stomach Burning, light headed +
Vomiting + Hot + cold spews
Post-lunch energy level: ⊘ low ○ medium ○ high

Dinner

Time: 6·15pm

List the foods you ate for dinner.

Fresh fish.

Actifry Chips

Tomato + Pepper Salad.

Cup of Tea with milk.

Choc Chip Cookie.

Drink Glass water
○ room-temp   ○ hot   ◉ cold

Drink _____
○ room-temp   ◉ hot   ○ cold

Comments: _____

Physical symptoms after meal: ○ **low**   ○ **intense**   ○ **non-existent**
○ Belching
○ Nausea
○ Stomach fullness or bloating
○ Upper abdominal pain and discomfort
○ Difficulty or pain with swallowing
○ Wheezing or dry cough

Other symptoms: Burning Stomach

Post-dinner energy level: ◉ low   ○ medium   ○ high

Snack

Time: 4·00

List the foods you ate as a snack.

_____

Drink Ginger lemon Tea   ○ room-temp   ◉ hot   ○ cold

Comments: To Try and ease Burning Sensation.

Post-snack energy level: ◉ low   ○ medium   ○ high

Snack

Time: 9·00

List the foods you ate as a snack.

_____

Drink Brandy + Port x2   ◉ room-temp   ○ hot   ○ cold

Comments: To help ease Burning Sensation.

Post-snack energy level: ○ low   ◉ medium   ○ high

Trigger points - milk + Low Fat Texan style Crisps

Medications & Supplements

Include prescription medication, over-the-counter medication & vitamin supplements.

1 Rennie -

1 Depression Tablet .

Energy level | Restfulness

Today's waking energy level?
● low　○ medium　○ high

# of times roused from sleep last night?
○ 1　○ 2　● 3+

Last night's reflux/GERD symptoms:

Bed raised?　○ Y　● N

Wedged Pillows?　● Y　○ N

Last meal time? 9.30

Approx bedtime? 11.00　am　(pm)

(Remember to give yourself at least 2-3 hours after meals before lying down.)

End-of-day notes

Noticeable change in symptoms? *(Ex: "Throat discomfort has completely disappeared.")*

Still Stomach Burn + hot, Dizziness has Dispersed a Bit

New terms to research

Books & websites with helpful info

Additional notes:

DATE 26th February

Breakfast

Time: 10:00

List the foods you ate for breakfast.

1 Slice of Toast with (1.30) Butter

1 hot Cross Bun with Butter- cup tea with milk

Drink Cup tea with milk
○ room-temp ○ hot ⊙ cold

Drink cup of Ginger + lemon Tea
○ room-temp ⊙ hot ○ cold

Comments: Felt alot Better this morning Just Tired.

Physical symptoms after meal: ○ **low** ○ **intense** ○ **non-existent**
○ Belching
○ Nausea
○ Stomach fullness or bloating
○ Upper abdominal pain and discomfort
○ Difficulty or pain with swallowing
○ Wheezing or dry cough

Other symptoms:

Post-breakfast energy level: ○ low ⊙ medium ○ high

Lunch

Time: 12:30

List the foods you ate for lunch.

Bowl of Chicken vegetable Soup, 1 yoghurt

Drink Glass water
○ room-temp ○ hot ⊙ cold

Drink
○ room-temp ○ hot ○ cold

Comments:

Physical symptoms after meal: ○ **low** ○ **intense** ⊙ **non-existent**
○ Belching
○ Nausea
○ Stomach fullness or bloating
○ Upper abdominal pain and discomfort
○ Difficulty or pain with swallowing
○ Wheezing or dry cough

Other symptoms:

Post-lunch energy level: ⊙ low ○ medium ○ high

Dinner

Time: 6:00 Pm

List the foods you ate for dinner.

lwsayna, Chips, Peas

_____

Drink _Cup of Tea with milk_   Drink _____
○ room-temp ⊘ hot ○ cold   ○ room-temp ○ hot ○ cold

Comments: _____

Physical symptoms after meal: ○ **low** ○ **intense** ⊘ **non-existent**
○ Belching   ○ Upper abdominal pain and discomfort
○ Nausea   ○ Difficulty or pain with swallowing
○ Stomach fullness or bloating   ○ Wheezing or dry cough

Other symptoms: None

Post-dinner energy level: ⊘ low ○ medium ○ high

Snack

Time: 3.30

List the foods you ate as a snack.

1 Banana, lcrenye

Drink _Guss water_   ○ room-temp ○ hot ⊘ cold

Comments: _____

Post-snack energy level: ⊘ low ○ medium ○ high

Snack

Time: 10.00

List the foods you ate as a snack.

Strawbery up cake

Drink _Tea with milk_   ○ room-temp ⊘ hot ○ cold

Comments: feel a slight Burning + Tummy Cramps

Post-snack energy level: ○ low ⊘ medium ○ high

Medications & Supplements

Include prescription medication, over-the-counter medication & vitamin supplements.

Depression Tablet

Vitimin B12

_____

_____

_____

Energy level | Restfulness

Today's waking energy level?
○ low ◉ medium ○ high

# of times roused from sleep last night?
◉ 1 ○ 2 ○ 3+

Last night's reflux/GERD symptoms:

_____

_____

Bed raised? ○ Y ◉ N

Wedged Pillows? ◉ Y ○ N

Last meal time? _10 oc_

Approx bedtime? _11.30_ am pm

(Remember to give yourself at least 2-3 hours after meals before lying down.)

End-of-day notes

Noticeable change in symptoms? *(Ex: "Throat discomfort has completely disappeared.")*

Burning getting Bad tonite again.

_____

New terms to research

_____

_____

Books & websites with helpful info

_____

_____

Additional notes:

_____

_____

_____

DATE	21th February 2014

Breakfast

Time: 8·00

List the foods you ate for breakfast.

~~2~~ 1 muffin Topped with

3 medullion of Bacon.

_____

🥤 **Drink** Cup Tea + milk!
○ room-temp ⦿ hot ○ cold

Drink _____
○ room-temp ○ hot ○ cold

Comments: Stomach a Bit Winny

Physical symptoms after meal: ⦿ low ○ intense ○ non-existent
○ Belching
○ Nausea
○ Stomach fullness or bloating
○ Upper abdominal pain and discomfort
○ Difficulty or pain with swallowing
○ Wheezing or dry cough

Other symptoms:

Post-breakfast energy level: ○ low ⦿ medium ○ high

Lunch

Time: _____

List the foods you ate for lunch.

Bowl of vegetable sup

Slice of Toast + Butter

1 fruit yoghurt

🥤 **Drink** Glass water
○ room-temp ○ hot ⦿ cold

Drink _____
○ room-temp ○ hot ○ cold

Comments:

Physical symptoms after meal: ⦿ low ○ intense ○ non-existent
○ Belching
○ Nausea
○ Stomach fullness or bloating
○ Upper abdominal pain and discomfort
○ Difficulty or pain with swallowing
○ Wheezing or dry cough

Other symptoms:

Post-lunch energy level: ○ low ⦿ medium ○ high

Dinner

Time: 6:00

List the foods you ate for dinner.

mince steak with
2 potatoes + carrots + peas.

1 choc-chip biscuit

Drink Glass water
○ room-temp ○ hot ⊘ cold

Drink Cup Tea + milk
○ room-temp ⊘ hot ○ cold

Comments:

Physical symptoms after meal: ○ **low** ○ **intense** ○ **non-existent**
- ○ Belching
- ○ Nausea
- ○ Stomach fullness or bloating
- ○ Upper abdominal pain and discomfort
- ○ Difficulty or pain with swallowing
- ○ Wheezing or dry cough

Other symptoms: No symptoms.

Post-dinner energy level: ○ low ○ medium ⊘ high

Snack

Time: 10:30

List the foods you ate as a snack.

1 Banana.

Drink Cup of Ginger + lemon Tea.
○ room-temp ⊘ hot ○ cold

Comments:

Post-snack energy level: ○ low ⊘ medium ○ high

Snack

Time: 10:00

List the foods you ate as a snack.

1 choc + caramel hot cross bun

Drink Tea with milk
○ room-temp ⊘ hot ○ cold

Comments:

Post-snack energy level: ○ low ○ medium ⊘ high

Medications & Supplements

Include prescription medication, over-the-counter medication & vitamin supplements.

O2morcie x2

UiTimin B12 x2

Depression Tablet

Energy level | Restfulness

Today's waking energy level?
○ low ⊘ medium ○ high

# of times roused from sleep last night?
⊘ 1   ○ 2   ○ 3+

Last night's reflux/GERD symptoms:

Bed raised?   ○ Y ⊘ N

Wedged Pillows?   ⊘ Y ○ N

Last meal time? 10:00 Pm

Approx bedtime? 11:00 am ⊘pm
(Remember to give yourself at least 2-3 hours after meals before lying down.)

End-of-day notes

Noticeable change in symptoms? *(Ex: "Throat discomfort has completely disappeared.")*

felt more eneugetic today

New terms to research

Books & websites with helpful info

Additional notes:

DATE	28th Febuary 2014

Breakfast

Time: _____

List the foods you ate for breakfast.

Slice of Tonst

with Butter

10:00

Choc + Carmel hot Cross Bun

with Butters

Drink Cup Tea with milk
○ room-temp ◉ hot ○ cold

Drink Ginger Tea.
○ room-temp ◉ hot ○ cold

Comments:

Physical symptoms after meal: ○ low ○ intense ◉ non-existent
- ○ Belching
- ○ Nausea
- ○ Stomach fullness or bloating
- ○ Upper abdominal pain and discomfort
- ○ Difficulty or pain with swallowing
- ○ Wheezing or dry cough

Other symptoms: Tired.

Post-breakfast energy level: ◉ low ○ medium ○ high

Lunch

Time: 3.30 pm

List the foods you ate for lunch.

2 Slices wht bread

with ham 1 yoghurt

mandarin orange

Drink Tea with milk
○ room-temp ○ hot ○ cold

Drink Glass water
○ room-temp ○ hot ○ cold

Comments:

Physical symptoms after meal: ○ low ○ intense ◉ non-existent
- ○ Belching
- ○ Nausea
- ○ Stomach fullness or bloating
- ○ Upper abdominal pain and discomfort
- ○ Difficulty or pain with swallowing
- ○ Wheezing or dry cough

Other symptoms:

Post-lunch energy level: ◉ low ○ medium ○ high

Dinner

Time: 6:00 pm

List the foods you ate for dinner.

2 Potatoes with
mince steak, carrot +
onion.

2 Sml mullums

Drink Glass Blackcurrant
○ room-temp   ○ hot   ⊘ cold

Drink Cup Tea with milk
○ room-temp   ⊘ hot   ○ cold

Comments:

Physical symptoms after meal: ○ **low**   ○ **intense**   ⊘ **non-existent**

○ Belching
○ Nausea
○ Stomach fullness or bloating

○ Upper abdominal pain and discomfort
○ Difficulty or pain with swallowing
○ Wheezing or dry cough

Other symptoms: limbs + Hips very sore

Post-dinner energy level: ○ low   ⊘ medium   ○ high

Snack

Time: 6:30 pm.

List the foods you ate as a snack.

hot Cross Bun + Butter

Drink Ginger Tea.   ○ room-temp   ⊘ hot   ○ cold

Comments:

Post-snack energy level: ⊘ low   ○ medium   ○ high

Snack

Time:

List the foods you ate as a snack.

Drink _____   ○ room-temp   ○ hot   ○ cold

Comments:

Post-snack energy level: ○ low   ○ medium   ○ high

Medications & Supplements

Include prescription medication, over-the-counter medication & vitamin supplements.

Depression Tablet

O2morole

Vitimin B12

_____

_____

Energy level | Restfulness

Today's waking energy level?
● low ○ medium ○ high

# of times roused from sleep last night?
● 1 ○ 2 ○ 3+

Last night's reflux/GERD symptoms:

_____

_____

Bed raised? ○ Y ● N

Wedged Pillows? ● Y ○ N

Last meal time? 10·30

Approx bedtime? 11·00 am pm

(Remember to give yourself at least 2-3 hours after meals before lying down.)

End-of-day notes

Noticeable change in symptoms? *(Ex: "Throat discomfort has completely disappeared.")*

Tingling Tongue

_____

New terms to research

Books & websites with helpful info

_____

_____

Additional notes:

_____

_____

_____

Breakfast

Time: 8:00

List the foods you ate for breakfast.

Unsliced Toasted

Sundaye muffin

_____

_____

_____

Drink Tea with milk
○ room-temp ● hot ○ cold

Drink _____
○ room-temp ○ hot ○ cold

Comments:

Physical symptoms after meal: ○ **low** ○ **intense** ● **non-existent**
○ Belching
○ Nausea
○ Stomach fullness or bloating
○ Upper abdominal pain and discomfort
○ Difficulty or pain with swallowing
○ Wheezing or dry cough

Other symptoms: Sore Bones + Hip.

Post-breakfast energy level: ○ low ● medium ○ high

Lunch

Time: 12:00

List the foods you ate for lunch.

2 Slices Wht Bread

with Butter filled with

Cooked Ham

mandarin orange

_____

_____

Drink Tea with milk
○ room-temp ● hot ○ cold

Drink _____
○ room-temp ○ hot ○ cold

Comments:

Physical symptoms after meal: ● **low** ○ **intense** ○ **non-existent**
○ Belching
○ Nausea
○ Stomach fullness or bloating
○ Upper abdominal pain and discomfort
○ Difficulty or pain with swallowing
○ Wheezing or dry cough

Other symptoms:

Post-lunch energy level: ○ low ● medium ○ high

Dinner
Time: 6:00

List the foods you ate for dinner.

Achry Chips with
mushrooms + Burger
Slice of Bread.

Drink Cup Tea with milk
○ room-temp ◉ hot ○ cold

Drink _____
○ room-temp ○ hot ○ cold

Comments: 1 Low Fat Bar

Physical symptoms after meal: ○ **low**   ○ **intense**   ◉ **non-existent**
- ○ Belching
- ○ Nausea
- ○ Stomach fullness or bloating
- ○ Upper abdominal pain and discomfort
- ○ Difficulty or pain with swallowing
- ○ Wheezing or dry cough

Other symptoms: Sore hip + Bones.

Post-dinner energy level: ◉ low   ○ medium   ○ high

Snack
Time: 10:30

List the foods you ate as a snack.

1 apple

Drink Cup Ginger Tea
○ room-temp   ◉ hot   ○ cold

Comments: _____

Post-snack energy level: ○ low   ◉ medium   ○ high

Snack
Time: 10:30

List the foods you ate as a snack.

Hot Cross Bun.

Drink Cup Tea with milk
○ room-temp   ◉ hot   ○ cold

Comments: Slight Burning

Post-snack energy level: ◉ low   ○ medium   ○ high

Medications & Supplements

Include prescription medication, over-the-counter medication & vitamin supplements.

Depression Pil

_____   _____

_____   _____

_____   _____

_____   _____

Energy level | Restfulness

Today's waking energy level?
◉ low ○ medium ○ high

# of times roused from sleep last night?
○ 1 ◉ 2 ○ 3+

Last night's reflux/GERD symptoms:

_____   _____

_____   _____

Bed raised? ○ Y ◉ N   Wedged Pillows? ◉ Y ○ N

Last meal time? _10.30_   Approx bedtime? _____ am pm
(Remember to give yourself at least 2-3 hours after meals before lying down.)

End-of-day notes

Noticeable change in symptoms? *(Ex: "Throat discomfort has completely disappeared.")*

_____

_____

New terms to research   Books & websites with helpful info

_____   _____

_____   _____

Additional notes:

_____

_____

_____

DATE	2nd March

Breakfast
Time: 9.00

List the foods you ate for breakfast.

2 Slices wht Bread

Toasted filled with Turkey.

_____

Drink Cup Tea + milk.
- ○ room-temp ● hot ○ cold

Drink _____
- ○ room-temp ○ hot ○ cold

Comments:

Physical symptoms after meal: ● low ○ intense ○ non-existent
- ○ Belching
- ○ Nausea
- ○ Stomach fullness or bloating
- ○ Upper abdominal pain and discomfort
- ○ Difficulty or pain with swallowing
- ○ Wheezing or dry cough

Other symptoms: No Symptoms today

Post-breakfast energy level: ○ low ○ medium ○ high

Lunch
Time: 2.30

List the foods you ate for lunch.

Bowl of soup with 2

Slices wholemeal Bread.

_____

Drink Cup Tea + milk.
- ○ room-temp ● hot ○ cold

Drink _____
- ○ room-temp ○ hot ○ cold

Comments:

Physical symptoms after meal: ○ low ○ intense ○ non-existent
- ○ Belching
- ○ Nausea
- ○ Stomach fullness or bloating
- ○ Upper abdominal pain and discomfort
- ○ Difficulty or pain with swallowing
- ○ Wheezing or dry cough

Other symptoms: No Symptoms

Post-lunch energy level: ○ low ● medium ○ high

Dinner

Time: 7.00

List the foods you ate for dinner.

Chicken Breast with

oven chips + Peas.

_____

Drink 2 cup merjans + orange
○ room-temp ○ hot ● cold

Drink _____
○ room-temp ○ hot ○ cold

Comments:

Physical symptoms after meal: ● low ○ intense ○ non-existent
○ Belching
○ Nausea
○ Stomach fullness or bloating
○ Upper abdominal pain and discomfort
○ Difficulty or pain with swallowing
○ Wheezing or dry cough

Other symptoms: No Symptoms

Post-dinner energy level: ○ low ● medium ○ high

Snack

Time: 3.00

List the foods you ate as a snack.

L.fat Choc Bar

Drink Cup Tea + milk.   ○ room-temp ● hot ○ cold

Comments:

Post-snack energy level: ○ low ○ medium ○ high

Snack

Time: _____

List the foods you ate as a snack.

PKT Peanuts

Drink No Drink   ○ room-temp ○ hot ○ cold

Comments:

Post-snack energy level: ○ low ● medium ○ high

Medications & Supplements

Include prescription medication, over-the-counter medication & vitamin supplements.

Depression Pill

_____   _____

_____   _____

_____   _____

_____   _____

Energy level | Restfulness

Today's waking energy level?
⊘ low   ○ medium   ○ high

# of times roused from sleep last night?
⊘ 1   ○ 2   ○ 3+

Last night's reflux/GERD symptoms:

None
_____   _____

_____   _____

Bed raised?   ⊘ Y   ○ N   Wedged Pillows?   ⊘ Y   ○ N

Last meal time? 10:00   Approx bedtime? 11:30   am   pm
(Remember to give yourself at least 2-3 hours after meals before lying down.)

End-of-day notes

Noticeable change in symptoms? _(Ex: "Throat discomfort has completely disappeared.")_

_____

_____

New terms to research   Books & websites with helpful info

_____   _____

_____   _____

Additional notes:

_____

_____

_____

DATE	Sunday 3rd March.

Breakfast

Time: 9-00

List the foods you ate for breakfast.

2 Slices whT Bread

Tursted fileed with Turkey

Drink Cup Tea + milk
○ room-temp ● hot ○ cold

Drink _____
○ room-temp ○ hot ○ cold

Comments:

Physical symptoms after meal: ○ **low** ○ **intense** ○ **non-existent**
○ Belching
○ Nausea
○ Stomach fullness or bloating
○ Upper abdominal pain and discomfort
○ Difficulty or pain with swallowing
○ Wheezing or dry cough

Other symptoms: No Sypmflems .

Post-breakfast energy level: ○ low ● medium ○ high

Lunch

Time: 2 00

List the foods you ate for lunch.

wBtr 2 small Rolls

fileed wuh Ham

Drink Cup Tea + milk.
○ room-temp ● hot ○ cold

Drink _____
○ room-temp ○ hot ○ cold

Comments:

Physical symptoms after meal: ○ **low** ○ **intense** ● **non-existent**
○ Belching
○ Nausea
○ Stomach fullness or bloating
○ Upper abdominal pain and discomfort
○ Difficulty or pain with swallowing
○ Wheezing or dry cough

Other symptoms:

Post-lunch energy level: ○ low ○ medium ● high

Dinner

Time: 430

List the foods you ate for dinner.

2 Roast Potatoes with lamb, Broclli + Runner Beans.

Ice cream + Jelly
1 Choc mallow

Drink _____
○ room-temp ○ hot ○ cold

Drink cup Tea with milk
○ room-temp ⦿ hot ○ cold

Comments: _____

Physical symptoms after meal: ⦿ low ○ intense ○ non-existent

○ Belching
○ Nausea
○ Stomach fullness or bloating

○ Upper abdominal pain and discomfort
○ Difficulty or pain with swallowing
○ Wheezing or dry cough

Other symptoms: Irritable Stomach.

Post-dinner energy level: ○ low ⦿ medium ○ high

Snack

Time: _____

List the foods you ate as a snack.

L.F Choc Bar

Drink cup Tea + milk.
○ room-temp ⦿ hot ○ cold

Comments: _____

Post-snack energy level: ○ low ⦿ medium ○ high

Snack

Time: _____

List the foods you ate as a snack.

12 Rice crackers.

Drink 1 Glass of Red wine ⦿ room-temp ○ hot ○ cold

Comments: _____

Post-snack energy level: ○ low ⦿ medium ○ high

Medications & Supplements

Include prescription medication, over-the-counter medication & vitamin supplements.

Depression Pill.

_____   _____

_____   _____

_____   _____

_____   _____

_____   _____

Energy level | Restfulness

Today's waking energy level?
○ low   ○ medium   Ⓞ high

# of times roused from sleep last night?
Ⓞ 1   ○ 2   ○ 3+

Last night's reflux/GERD symptoms:

_____   _____

_____   _____

Bed raised?   ○ Y Ⓞ N   Wedged Pillows? Ⓞ Y ○ N

Last meal time? ~~too~~ 8:00   Approx bedtime? 10:00 am pm
(Remember to give yourself at least 2-3 hours after meals before lying down.)

End-of-day notes

Noticeable change in symptoms? _(Ex: "Throat discomfort has completely disappeared.")_

A Slight Burning, Irritable Stomach + Tired.

_____

New terms to research   Books & websites with helpful info

_____   _____

_____   _____

Additional notes:

2 walks Today
Felt much Better after a walk.

_____

Breakfast   Time: _____

List the foods you ate for breakfast.

_____   _____

_____   _____

_____   _____

Drink _____   **Drink** _____
○ room-temp   ○ hot   ○ cold   ○ room-temp   ○ hot   ○ cold

Comments: _____

Physical symptoms after meal: ○ **low**   ○ **intense**   ○ **non-existent**
○ Belching   ○ Upper abdominal pain and discomfort
○ Nausea   ○ Difficulty or pain with swallowing
○ Stomach fullness or bloating   ○ Wheezing or dry cough

Other symptoms: _____

Post-breakfast energy level: ○ low   ○ medium   ○ high

Lunch   Time: _____

List the foods you ate for lunch.

_____   _____

_____   _____

_____   _____

Drink _____   **Drink** _____
○ room-temp   ○ hot   ○ cold   ○ room-temp   ○ hot   ○ cold

Comments: _____

Physical symptoms after meal: ○ **low**   ○ **intense**   ○ **non-existent**
○ Belching   ○ Upper abdominal pain and discomfort
○ Nausea   ○ Difficulty or pain with swallowing
○ Stomach fullness or bloating   ○ Wheezing or dry cough

Other symptoms: _____

Post-lunch energy level: ○ low   ○ medium   ○ high

Dinner

Time: _____

List the foods you ate for dinner.

_____   _____

_____   _____

_____   _____

Drink _____   **Drink** _____
○ room-temp   ○ hot   ○ cold   ○ room-temp   ○ hot   ○ cold

Physical symptoms after meal: ○ **low**   ○ **intense**   ○ **non-existent**

○ Belching   ○ Upper abdominal pain and discomfort
○ Nausea   ○ Difficulty or pain with swallowing
○ Stomach fullness or bloating   ○ Wheezing or dry cough

Other symptoms: _____

Post-dinner energy level: ○ low   ○ medium   ○ high

Snack

Time: _____

List the foods you ate as a snack.

_____   _____

Drink _____   ○ room-temp   ○ hot   ○ cold

Comments: _____

Post-snack energy level: ○ low   ○ medium   ○ high

Snack

Time: _____

List the foods you ate as a snack.

_____   _____

Drink _____   ○ room-temp   ○ hot   ○ cold

Comments: _____

Post-snack energy level: ○ low   ○ medium   ○ high

Medications & Supplements

Include prescription medication, over-the-counter medication & vitamin supplements.

_____   _____

_____   _____

_____   _____

_____   _____

_____   _____

Energy level | Restfulness

Today's waking energy level?
○ low   ○ medium   ○ high

# of times roused from sleep last night?
○ 1   ○ 2   ○ 3+

Last night's reflux/GERD symptoms:

_____   _____

_____   _____

Bed raised?   ○ Y   ○ N   Wedged Pillows?   ○ Y   ○ N

Last meal time? _____   Approx bedtime? _____   am   pm
(Remember to give yourself at least 2-3 hours after meals before lying down.)

End-of-day notes

Noticeable change in symptoms? *(Ex: "Throat discomfort has completely disappeared.")*

_____

_____

New terms to research   Books & websites with helpful info

_____   _____

_____   _____

Additional notes:

_____

_____

_____

Breakfast   Time: _____

List the foods you ate for breakfast.

_____   _____

_____   _____

Drink _____   **Drink** _____
○ room-temp   ○ hot   ○ cold   ○ room-temp   ○ hot   ○ cold

Comments: _____

Physical symptoms after meal: ○ **low**   ○ **intense**   ○ **non-existent**
○ Belching   ○ Upper abdominal pain and discomfort
○ Nausea   ○ Difficulty or pain with swallowing
○ Stomach fullness or bloating ○ Wheezing or dry cough

Other symptoms: _____

Post-breakfast energy level: ○ low   ○ medium   ○ high

Lunch   Time: _____

List the foods you ate for lunch.

_____   _____

_____   _____

Drink _____   **Drink** _____
○ room-temp   ○ hot   ○ cold   ○ room-temp   ○ hot   ○ cold

Comments: _____

Physical symptoms after meal: ○ **low**   ○ **intense**   ○ **non-existent**
○ Belching   ○ Upper abdominal pain and discomfort
○ Nausea   ○ Difficulty or pain with swallowing
○ Stomach fullness or bloating ○ Wheezing or dry cough

Other symptoms: _____

Post-lunch energy level: ○ low   ○ medium   ○ high

Dinner

Time: _____

List the foods you ate for dinner.

_____   _____

_____   _____

_____   _____

Drink _____   **Drink** _____
○ room-temp   ○ hot   ○ cold   ○ room-temp   ○ hot   ○ cold

Comments:

Physical symptoms after meal: ○ **low**   ○ **intense**   ○ **non-existent**
○ Belching   ○ Upper abdominal pain and discomfort
○ Nausea   ○ Difficulty or pain with swallowing
○ Stomach fullness or bloating   ○ Wheezing or dry cough

Other symptoms:

Post-dinner energy level: ○ low   ○ medium   ○ high

Snack

Time: _____

List the foods you ate as a snack.

_____   _____

Drink _____   ○ room-temp   ○ hot   ○ cold

Comments:

Post-snack energy level: ○ low   ○ medium   ○ high

Snack

Time: _____

List the foods you ate as a snack.

_____   _____

Drink _____   ○ room-temp   ○ hot   ○ cold

Comments:

Post-snack energy level: ○ low   ○ medium   ○ high

Medications & Supplements

Include prescription medication, over-the-counter medication & vitamin supplements.

_____   _____

_____   _____

_____   _____

_____   _____

Energy level | Restfulness

Today's waking energy level?
○ low   ○ medium   ○ high

# of times roused from sleep last night?
○ 1   ○ 2   ○ 3+

Last night's reflux/GERD symptoms:

_____   _____

_____   _____

Bed raised?   ○ Y   ○ N   Wedged Pillows?   ○ Y   ○ N

Last meal time? _____   Approx bedtime? _____   am   pm
(Remember to give yourself at least 2-3 hours after meals before lying down.)

End-of-day notes

Noticeable change in symptoms? _(Ex: "Throat discomfort has completely disappeared.")_

_____

_____

New terms to research   Books & websites with helpful info

_____   _____

_____   _____

Additional notes:

_____

_____

_____

Breakfast
Time: _____

List the foods you ate for breakfast.

_____   _____

_____   _____

_____   _____

Drink _____   **Drink** _____
○ room-temp   ○ hot   ○ cold   ○ room-temp   ○ hot   ○ cold

Comments:

Physical symptoms after meal: ○ **low**   ○ **intense**   ○ **non-existent**
○ Belching   ○ Upper abdominal pain and discomfort
○ Nausea   ○ Difficulty or pain with swallowing
○ Stomach fullness or bloating   ○ Wheezing or dry cough

Other symptoms:

Post-breakfast energy level: ○ low   ○ medium   ○ high

Lunch
Time: _____

List the foods you ate for lunch.

_____   _____

_____   _____

_____   _____

Drink _____   **Drink** _____
○ room-temp   ○ hot   ○ cold   ○ room-temp   ○ hot   ○ cold

Comments:

Physical symptoms after meal: ○ **low**   ○ **intense**   ○ **non-existent**
○ Belching   ○ Upper abdominal pain and discomfort
○ Nausea   ○ Difficulty or pain with swallowing
○ Stomach fullness or bloating   ○ Wheezing or dry cough

Other symptoms:

Post-lunch energy level: ○ low   ○ medium   ○ high

Dinner

Time: _____

List the foods you ate for dinner.

_____   _____

_____   _____

_____   _____

Drink _____   **Drink** _____
○ room-temp ○ hot ○ cold   ○ room-temp ○ hot ○ cold

Comments:

Physical symptoms after meal: ○ **low**   ○ **intense**   ○ **non-existent**
○ Belching   ○ Upper abdominal pain and discomfort
○ Nausea   ○ Difficulty or pain with swallowing
○ Stomach fullness or bloating   ○ Wheezing or dry cough

Other symptoms:

Post-dinner energy level: ○ low   ○ medium   ○ high

Snack

Time: _____

List the foods you ate as a snack.

_____   _____

Drink _____   ○ room-temp   ○ hot   ○ cold

Comments:

Post-snack energy level: ○ low   ○ medium   ○ high

Snack

Time: _____

List the foods you ate as a snack.

_____   _____

Drink _____   ○ room-temp   ○ hot   ○ cold

Comments:

Post-snack energy level: ○ low   ○ medium   ○ high

Medications & Supplements

Include prescription medication, over-the-counter medication & vitamin supplements.

_____   _____

_____   _____

_____   _____

_____   _____

_____   _____

Energy level | Restfulness

Today's waking energy level?
○ low   ○ medium   ○ high

# of times roused from sleep last night?
○ 1   ○ 2   ○ 3+

Last night's reflux/GERD symptoms:

_____   _____

_____   _____

Bed raised?   ○ Y   ○ N   Wedged Pillows?   ○ Y   ○ N

Last meal time? _____   Approx bedtime? _____   am   pm
(Remember to give yourself at least 2-3 hours after meals before lying down.)

End-of-day notes

Noticeable change in symptoms? _(Ex: "Throat discomfort has completely disappeared.")_

_____

_____

New terms to research   Books & websites with helpful info

_____   _____

_____   _____

Additional notes:

_____

_____

_____

Breakfast

Time: _____

List the foods you ate for breakfast.

_____   _____

_____   _____

_____   _____

Drink _____   **Drink** _____
  ○ room-temp ○ hot ○ cold   ○ room-temp ○ hot ○ cold

Comments: _____

Physical symptoms after meal: ○ **low** ○ **intense** ○ **non-existent**
○ Belching   ○ Upper abdominal pain and discomfort
○ Nausea   ○ Difficulty or pain with swallowing
○ Stomach fullness or bloating   ○ Wheezing or dry cough

Other symptoms: _____

Post-breakfast energy level: ○ low ○ medium ○ high

Lunch

Time: _____

List the foods you ate for lunch.

_____   _____

_____   _____

_____   _____

Drink _____   **Drink** _____
  ○ room-temp ○ hot ○ cold   ○ room-temp ○ hot ○ cold

Comments: _____

Physical symptoms after meal: ○ **low** ○ **intense** ○ **non-existent**
○ Belching   ○ Upper abdominal pain and discomfort
○ Nausea   ○ Difficulty or pain with swallowing
○ Stomach fullness or bloating   ○ Wheezing or dry cough

Other symptoms: _____

Post-lunch energy level: ○ low ○ medium ○ high

Dinner

Time: _____

List the foods you ate for dinner.

_____   _____

_____   _____

_____   _____

Drink _____   **Drink** _____
○ room-temp ○ hot ○ cold   ○ room-temp ○ hot ○ cold

Comments: _____

Physical symptoms after meal: ○ **low** ○ **intense** ○ **non-existent**
○ Belching   ○ Upper abdominal pain and discomfort
○ Nausea   ○ Difficulty or pain with swallowing
○ Stomach fullness or bloating   ○ Wheezing or dry cough

Other symptoms: _____

Post-dinner energy level: ○ low ○ medium ○ high

Snack

Time: _____

List the foods you ate as a snack.

_____   _____

Drink _____   ○ room-temp ○ hot ○ cold

Comments: _____

Post-snack energy level: ○ low ○ medium ○ high

Snack

Time: _____

List the foods you ate as a snack.

_____   _____

Drink _____   ○ room-temp ○ hot ○ cold

Comments: _____

Post-snack energy level: ○ low ○ medium ○ high

Medications & Supplements

Include prescription medication, over-the-counter medication & vitamin supplements.

_____   _____

_____   _____

_____   _____

_____   _____

_____   _____

Energy level | Restfulness

Today's waking energy level?
○ low   ○ medium   ○ high

# of times roused from sleep last night?
○ 1   ○ 2   ○ 3+

Last night's reflux/GERD symptoms:

_____   _____

_____   _____

Bed raised?   ○ Y   ○ N   Wedged Pillows?   ○ Y   ○ N

Last meal time? _____   Approx bedtime? _____ am pm
(Remember to give yourself at least 2-3 hours after meals before lying down.)

End-of-day notes

Noticeable change in symptoms? _(Ex: "Throat discomfort has completely disappeared.")_

_____

_____

New terms to research   Books & websites with helpful info

_____   _____

_____   _____

Additional notes:

_____

_____

_____

DATE	

Breakfast   Time: _____

List the foods you ate for breakfast.

_____   _____

_____   _____

_____   _____

Drink _____   **Drink** _____
○ room-temp ○ hot ○ cold   ○ room-temp ○ hot ○ cold

Comments: _____

Physical symptoms after meal: ○ **low**   ○ **intense**   ○ **non-existent**
○ Belching   ○ Upper abdominal pain and discomfort
○ Nausea   ○ Difficulty or pain with swallowing
○ Stomach fullness or bloating   ○ Wheezing or dry cough

Other symptoms: _____

Post-breakfast energy level: ○ low ○ medium ○ high

Lunch   Time: _____

List the foods you ate for lunch.

_____   _____

_____   _____

_____   _____

Drink _____   **Drink** _____
○ room-temp ○ hot ○ cold   ○ room-temp ○ hot ○ cold

Comments: _____

Physical symptoms after meal: ○ **low**   ○ **intense**   ○ **non-existent**
○ Belching   ○ Upper abdominal pain and discomfort
○ Nausea   ○ Difficulty or pain with swallowing
○ Stomach fullness or bloating   ○ Wheezing or dry cough

Other symptoms: _____

Post-lunch energy level: ○ low ○ medium ○ high

Dinner

Time: _____

List the foods you ate for dinner.

_____   _____

_____   _____

_____   _____

Drink _____   **Drink** _____
○ room-temp ○ hot ○ cold   ○ room-temp ○ hot ○ cold

Comments: _____

Physical symptoms after meal: ○ **low** ○ **intense** ○ **non-existent**
○ Belching   ○ Upper abdominal pain and discomfort
○ Nausea   ○ Difficulty or pain with swallowing
○ Stomach fullness or bloating   ○ Wheezing or dry cough

Other symptoms: _____

Post-dinner energy level: ○ low ○ medium ○ high

Snack

Time: _____

List the foods you ate as a snack.

_____   _____

Drink _____   ○ room-temp ○ hot ○ cold

Comments: _____

Post-snack energy level: ○ low ○ medium ○ high

Snack

Time: _____

List the foods you ate as a snack.

_____   _____

Drink _____   ○ room-temp ○ hot ○ cold

Comments: _____

Post-snack energy level: ○ low ○ medium ○ high

Medications & Supplements

Include prescription medication, over-the-counter medication & vitamin supplements.

_____   _____

_____   _____

_____   _____

_____   _____

_____   _____

Energy level | Restfulness

Today's waking energy level?
○ low   ○ medium   ○ high

# of times roused from sleep last night?
○ 1   ○ 2   ○ 3+

Last night's reflux/GERD symptoms:

_____   _____

_____   _____

Bed raised?   ○ Y   ○ N   Wedged Pillows?   ○ Y   ○ N

Last meal time? _____   Approx bedtime? _____ am   pm

(Remember to give yourself at least 2-3 hours after meals before lying down.)

End-of-day notes

Noticeable change in symptoms? *(Ex: "Throat discomfort has completely disappeared.")*

_____

_____

New terms to research   Books & websites with helpful info

_____   _____

_____   _____

Additional notes:

_____

_____

_____

Breakfast   Time: _____

List the foods you ate for breakfast.

_____   _____

_____   _____

_____   _____

Drink _____   **Drink** _____
○ room-temp   ○ hot   ○ cold   ○ room-temp   ○ hot   ○ cold

Comments: _____

Physical symptoms after meal: ○ **low**   ○ **intense**   ○ **non-existent**
○ Belching   ○ Upper abdominal pain and discomfort
○ Nausea   ○ Difficulty or pain with swallowing
○ Stomach fullness or bloating   ○ Wheezing or dry cough

Other symptoms: _____

Post-breakfast energy level: ○ low   ○ medium   ○ high

Lunch   Time: _____

List the foods you ate for lunch.

_____   _____

_____   _____

_____   _____

Drink _____   **Drink** _____
○ room-temp   ○ hot   ○ cold   ○ room-temp   ○ hot   ○ cold

Comments: _____

Physical symptoms after meal: ○ **low**   ○ **intense**   ○ **non-existent**
○ Belching   ○ Upper abdominal pain and discomfort
○ Nausea   ○ Difficulty or pain with swallowing
○ Stomach fullness or bloating   ○ Wheezing or dry cough

Other symptoms: _____

Post-lunch energy level: ○ low   ○ medium   ○ high

Dinner

Time: _____

List the foods you ate for dinner.

_____   _____

_____   _____

_____   _____

Drink _____   **Drink** _____

○ room-temp   ○ hot   ○ cold   ○ room-temp   ○ hot   ○ cold

Comments: _____

Physical symptoms after meal: ○ **low**   ○ **intense**   ○ **non-existent**

○ Belching   ○ Upper abdominal pain and discomfort

○ Nausea   ○ Difficulty or pain with swallowing

○ Stomach fullness or bloating   ○ Wheezing or dry cough

Other symptoms: _____

Post-dinner energy level: ○ low   ○ medium   ○ high

Snack

Time: _____

List the foods you ate as a snack.

_____   _____

Drink _____   ○ room-temp   ○ hot   ○ cold

Comments: _____

Post-snack energy level: ○ low   ○ medium   ○ high

Snack

Time: _____

List the foods you ate as a snack.

_____   _____

Drink _____   ○ room-temp   ○ hot   ○ cold

Comments: _____

Post-snack energy level: ○ low   ○ medium   ○ high

Medications & Supplements

Include prescription medication, over-the-counter medication & vitamin supplements.

_____   _____

_____   _____

_____   _____

_____   _____

_____   _____

Energy level | Restfulness

Today's waking energy level?
○ low   ○ medium   ○ high

# of times roused from sleep last night?
○ 1   ○ 2   ○ 3+

Last night's reflux/GERD symptoms:

_____   _____

_____   _____

Bed raised?   ○ Y   ○ N   Wedged Pillows?   ○ Y   ○ N

Last meal time? _____   Approx bedtime? _____   am   pm
(Remember to give yourself at least 2-3 hours after meals before lying down.)

End-of-day notes

Noticeable change in symptoms? _(Ex: "Throat discomfort has completely disappeared.")_

_____

_____

New terms to research   Books & websites with helpful info

_____   _____

_____   _____

Additional notes:

_____

_____

_____

Breakfast   Time: _____

List the foods you ate for breakfast.

_____   _____

_____   _____

_____   _____

Drink _____   **Drink** _____
○ room-temp   ○ hot   ○ cold   ○ room-temp   ○ hot   ○ cold

Comments:
_____

Physical symptoms after meal: ○ **low**   ○ **intense**   ○ **non-existent**
○ Belching   ○ Upper abdominal pain and discomfort
○ Nausea   ○ Difficulty or pain with swallowing
○ Stomach fullness or bloating   ○ Wheezing or dry cough

Other symptoms:
_____

Post-breakfast energy level: ○ low   ○ medium   ○ high

Lunch   Time: _____

List the foods you ate for lunch.

_____   _____

_____   _____

_____   _____

Drink _____   **Drink** _____
○ room-temp   ○ hot   ○ cold   ○ room-temp   ○ hot   ○ cold

Comments:
_____

Physical symptoms after meal: ○ **low**   ○ **intense**   ○ **non-existent**
○ Belching   ○ Upper abdominal pain and discomfort
○ Nausea   ○ Difficulty or pain with swallowing
○ Stomach fullness or bloating   ○ Wheezing or dry cough

Other symptoms:
_____

Post-lunch energy level: ○ low   ○ medium   ○ high

Dinner

Time: _____

List the foods you ate for dinner.

_____   _____

_____   _____

_____   _____

Drink _____   **Drink** _____
○ room-temp ○ hot ○ cold   ○ room-temp ○ hot ○ cold

_____

Physical symptoms after meal: ○ **low** ○ **intense** ○ **non-existent**
○ Belching   ○ Upper abdominal pain and discomfort
○ Nausea   ○ Difficulty or pain with swallowing
○ Stomach fullness or bloating ○ Wheezing or dry cough

Other symptoms: _____

Post-dinner energy level: ○ low ○ medium ○ high

Snack

Time: _____

List the foods you ate as a snack.

_____   _____

Drink _____   ○ room-temp ○ hot ○ cold

Comments: _____

Post-snack energy level: ○ low ○ medium ○ high

Snack

Time: _____

List the foods you ate as a snack.

_____   _____

Drink _____   ○ room-temp ○ hot ○ cold

Comments: _____

Post-snack energy level: ○ low ○ medium ○ high

Medications & Supplements

Include prescription medication, over-the-counter medication & vitamin supplements.

_____   _____

_____   _____

_____   _____

_____   _____

_____   _____

Energy level | Restfulness

Today's waking energy level?
○ low   ○ medium   ○ high

# of times roused from sleep last night?
○ 1   ○ 2   ○ 3+

Last night's reflux/GERD symptoms:

_____   _____

_____   _____

Bed raised?   ○ Y   ○ N   Wedged Pillows?   ○ Y   ○ N

Last meal time? _____   Approx bedtime? _____ am   pm
(Remember to give yourself at least 2-3 hours after meals before lying down.)

End-of-day notes

Noticeable change in symptoms? *(Ex: "Throat discomfort has completely disappeared.")*

_____

_____

New terms to research   Books & websites with helpful info

_____   _____

_____   _____

Additional notes:

_____

_____

_____

Breakfast

Time: _____

List the foods you ate for breakfast.

_____   _____

_____   _____

_____   _____

Drink _____   **Drink** _____
○ room-temp   ○ hot   ○ cold   ○ room-temp   ○ hot   ○ cold

Comments:

Physical symptoms after meal: ○ **low**   ○ **intense**   ○ **non-existent**
○ Belching   ○ Upper abdominal pain and discomfort
○ Nausea   ○ Difficulty or pain with swallowing
○ Stomach fullness or bloating ○ Wheezing or dry cough

Other symptoms:

Post-breakfast energy level: ○ low   ○ medium   ○ high

Lunch

Time: _____

List the foods you ate for lunch.

_____   _____

_____   _____

_____   _____

Drink _____   **Drink** _____
○ room-temp   ○ hot   ○ cold   ○ room-temp   ○ hot   ○ cold

Comments:

Physical symptoms after meal: ○ **low**   ○ **intense**   ○ **non-existent**
○ Belching   ○ Upper abdominal pain and discomfort
○ Nausea   ○ Difficulty or pain with swallowing
○ Stomach fullness or bloating ○ Wheezing or dry cough

Other symptoms:

Post-lunch energy level: ○ low   ○ medium   ○ high

Dinner

Time: _____

List the foods you ate for dinner.

_____   _____

_____   _____

_____   _____

Drink _____   **Drink** _____
○ room-temp ○ hot ○ cold   ○ room-temp ○ hot ○ cold

Comments:
_____

Physical symptoms after meal: ○ **low** ○ **intense** ○ **non-existent**
○ Belching   ○ Upper abdominal pain and discomfort
○ Nausea   ○ Difficulty or pain with swallowing
○ Stomach fullness or bloating ○ Wheezing or dry cough

Other symptoms: _____

Post-dinner energy level: ○ low ○ medium ○ high

Snack

Time: _____

List the foods you ate as a snack.

_____   _____

Drink _____ ○ room-temp ○ hot ○ cold

Comments: _____

Post-snack energy level: ○ low ○ medium ○ high

Snack

Time: _____

List the foods you ate as a snack.

_____   _____

Drink _____ ○ room-temp ○ hot ○ cold

Comments: _____

Post-snack energy level: ○ low ○ medium ○ high

Medications & Supplements

Include prescription medication, over-the-counter medication & vitamin supplements.

_____   _____

_____   _____

_____   _____

_____   _____

_____   _____

Energy level | Restfulness

Today's waking energy level?
○ low   ○ medium   ○ high

# of times roused from sleep last night?
○ 1   ○ 2   ○ 3+

Last night's reflux/GERD symptoms:

_____   _____

_____   _____

Bed raised?   ○ Y   ○ N   Wedged Pillows?   ○ Y   ○ N

Last meal time? _____   Approx bedtime? _____ am pm
(Remember to give yourself at least 2-3 hours after meals before lying down.)

End-of-day notes

Noticeable change in symptoms? *(Ex: "Throat discomfort has completely disappeared.")*

_____

_____

New terms to research   Books & websites with helpful info

_____   _____

_____   _____

Additional notes:

_____

_____

_____

Breakfast
Time: _____

List the foods you ate for breakfast.

_____   _____

_____   _____

_____   _____

Drink _____   **Drink** _____
  ○ room-temp   ○ hot   ○ cold   ○ room-temp   ○ hot   ○ cold

Comments:

Physical symptoms after meal: ○ **low**   ○ **intense**   ○ **non-existent**
○ Belching   ○ Upper abdominal pain and discomfort
○ Nausea   ○ Difficulty or pain with swallowing
○ Stomach fullness or bloating   ○ Wheezing or dry cough

Other symptoms:

Post-breakfast energy level: ○ low   ○ medium   ○ high

Lunch
Time: _____

List the foods you ate for lunch.

_____   _____

_____   _____

_____   _____

Drink _____   **Drink** _____
  ○ room-temp   ○ hot   ○ cold   ○ room-temp   ○ hot   ○ cold

Comments:

Physical symptoms after meal: ○ **low**   ○ **intense**   ○ **non-existent**
○ Belching   ○ Upper abdominal pain and discomfort
○ Nausea   ○ Difficulty or pain with swallowing
○ Stomach fullness or bloating   ○ Wheezing or dry cough

Other symptoms:

Post-lunch energy level: ○ low   ○ medium   ○ high

Dinner

Time: _____

List the foods you ate for dinner.

_____   _____

_____   _____

_____   _____

Drink _____   **Drink** _____
○ room-temp   ○ hot   ○ cold   ○ room-temp   ○ hot   ○ cold

Comments:

Physical symptoms after meal: ○ **low**   ○ **intense**   ○ **non-existent**
○ Belching   ○ Upper abdominal pain and discomfort
○ Nausea   ○ Difficulty or pain with swallowing
○ Stomach fullness or bloating   ○ Wheezing or dry cough

Other symptoms:

Post-dinner energy level: ○ low   ○ medium   ○ high

Snack

Time: _____

List the foods you ate as a snack.

_____   _____

Drink _____   ○ room-temp   ○ hot   ○ cold

Comments:

Post-snack energy level: ○ low   ○ medium   ○ high

Snack

Time: _____

List the foods you ate as a snack.

_____   _____

Drink _____   ○ room-temp   ○ hot   ○ cold

Comments:

Post-snack energy level: ○ low   ○ medium   ○ high

Medications & Supplements

Include prescription medication, over-the-counter medication & vitamin supplements.

_____   _____

_____   _____

_____   _____

_____   _____

_____   _____

Energy level | Restfulness

Today's waking energy level?
○ low   ○ medium   ○ high

# of times roused from sleep last night?
○ 1   ○ 2   ○ 3+

Last night's reflux/GERD symptoms:

_____   _____

_____   _____

Bed raised?   ○ Y   ○ N   Wedged Pillows?   ○ Y   ○ N

Last meal time? _____   Approx bedtime? _____ am pm
(Remember to give yourself at least 2-3 hours after meals before lying down.)

End-of-day notes

Noticeable change in symptoms? _(Ex: "Throat discomfort has completely disappeared.")_

_____

_____

New terms to research   Books & websites with helpful info

_____   _____

_____   _____

Additional notes:

_____

_____

_____

Breakfast   Time: _____

List the foods you ate for breakfast.

_____   _____

_____   _____

Drink _____   **Drink** _____
  ○ room-temp ○ hot ○ cold   ○ room-temp ○ hot ○ cold

Comments: _____

Physical symptoms after meal: ○ **low** ○ **intense** ○ **non-existent**

○ Belching   ○ Upper abdominal pain and discomfort
○ Nausea   ○ Difficulty or pain with swallowing
○ Stomach fullness or bloating   ○ Wheezing or dry cough

Other symptoms: _____

Post-breakfast energy level: ○ low ○ medium ○ high

Lunch   Time: _____

List the foods you ate for lunch.

_____   _____

_____   _____

Drink _____   **Drink** _____
  ○ room-temp ○ hot ○ cold   ○ room-temp ○ hot ○ cold

Comments: _____

Physical symptoms after meal: ○ **low** ○ **intense** ○ **non-existent**

○ Belching   ○ Upper abdominal pain and discomfort
○ Nausea   ○ Difficulty or pain with swallowing
○ Stomach fullness or bloating   ○ Wheezing or dry cough

Other symptoms: _____

Post-lunch energy level: ○ low ○ medium ○ high

Dinner

Time: _____

List the foods you ate for dinner.

_____   _____

_____   _____

_____   _____

Drink _____   **Drink** _____
    ○ room-temp ○ hot ○ cold   ○ room-temp ○ hot ○ cold

Comments:

Physical symptoms after meal: ○ **low** ○ **intense** ○ **non-existent**
○ Belching   ○ Upper abdominal pain and discomfort
○ Nausea   ○ Difficulty or pain with swallowing
○ Stomach fullness or bloating ○ Wheezing or dry cough

Other symptoms:

Post-dinner energy level: ○ low ○ medium ○ high

Snack

Time: _____

List the foods you ate as a snack.

_____   _____

Drink _____ ○ room-temp ○ hot ○ cold

Comments: _____

Post-snack energy level: ○ low ○ medium ○ high

Snack

Time: _____

List the foods you ate as a snack.

_____   _____

Drink _____ ○ room-temp ○ hot ○ cold

Comments: _____

Post-snack energy level: ○ low ○ medium ○ high

Medications & Supplements

Include prescription medication, over-the-counter medication & vitamin supplements.

_____   _____

_____   _____

_____   _____

_____   _____

_____   _____

Energy level | Restfulness

Today's waking energy level?
○ low   ○ medium   ○ high

# of times roused from sleep last night?
○ 1   ○ 2   ○ 3+

Last night's reflux/GERD symptoms:

_____   _____

_____   _____

Bed raised?   ○ Y   ○ N   Wedged Pillows?   ○ Y   ○ N

Last meal time? _____   Approx bedtime? _____   am   pm

(Remember to give yourself at least 2-3 hours after meals before lying down.)

End-of-day notes

Noticeable change in symptoms? *(Ex: "Throat discomfort has completely disappeared.")*

_____

_____

New terms to research   Books & websites with helpful info

_____   _____

_____   _____

Additional notes:

_____

_____

_____

Breakfast

Time: _____

List the foods you ate for breakfast.

_____   _____

_____   _____

_____   _____

Drink _____   **Drink** _____
○ room-temp   ○ hot   ○ cold   ○ room-temp   ○ hot   ○ cold

Comments: _____

Physical symptoms after meal: ○ **low**   ○ **intense**   ○ **non-existent**
○ Belching   ○ Upper abdominal pain and discomfort
○ Nausea   ○ Difficulty or pain with swallowing
○ Stomach fullness or bloating   ○ Wheezing or dry cough

Other symptoms: _____

Post-breakfast energy level: ○ low   ○ medium   ○ high

Lunch

Time: _____

List the foods you ate for lunch.

_____   _____

_____   _____

_____   _____

Drink _____   **Drink** _____
○ room-temp   ○ hot   ○ cold   ○ room-temp   ○ hot   ○ cold

Comments: _____

Physical symptoms after meal: ○ **low**   ○ **intense**   ○ **non-existent**
○ Belching   ○ Upper abdominal pain and discomfort
○ Nausea   ○ Difficulty or pain with swallowing
○ Stomach fullness or bloating   ○ Wheezing or dry cough

Other symptoms: _____

Post-lunch energy level: ○ low   ○ medium   ○ high

Dinner

Time: _____

List the foods you ate for dinner.

_____   _____

_____   _____

_____   _____

Drink _____   **Drink** _____
  ○ room-temp ○ hot ○ cold   ○ room-temp ○ hot ○ cold

Comments:

Physical symptoms after meal: ○ **low**   ○ **intense**   ○ **non-existent**
- ○ Belching
- ○ Nausea
- ○ Stomach fullness or bloating
- ○ Upper abdominal pain and discomfort
- ○ Difficulty or pain with swallowing
- ○ Wheezing or dry cough

Other symptoms:

Post-dinner energy level: ○ low   ○ medium   ○ high

Snack

Time: _____

List the foods you ate as a snack.

_____   _____

Drink _____   ○ room-temp   ○ hot   ○ cold

Comments:

Post-snack energy level: ○ low   ○ medium   ○ high

Snack

Time: _____

List the foods you ate as a snack.

_____   _____

Drink _____   ○ room-temp   ○ hot   ○ cold

Comments:

Post-snack energy level: ○ low   ○ medium   ○ high

Medications & Supplements

Include prescription medication, over-the-counter medication & vitamin supplements.

_____   _____

_____   _____

_____   _____

_____   _____

_____   _____

Energy level | Restfulness

Today's waking energy level?
○ low   ○ medium   ○ high

# of times roused from sleep last night?
○ 1   ○ 2   ○ 3+

Last night's reflux/GERD symptoms:

_____   _____

_____   _____

Bed raised?   ○ Y   ○ N   Wedged Pillows?   ○ Y   ○ N

Last meal time? _____   Approx bedtime? _____ am pm

(Remember to give yourself at least 2-3 hours after meals before lying down.)

End-of-day notes

Noticeable change in symptoms? *(Ex: "Throat discomfort has completely disappeared.")*

_____

_____

New terms to research   Books & websites with helpful info

_____   _____

_____   _____

Additional notes:

_____

_____

_____

Breakfast   Time: _____

List the foods you ate for breakfast.

_____   _____

_____   _____

_____   _____

Drink _____   **Drink** _____
○ room-temp ○ hot ○ cold   ○ room-temp ○ hot ○ cold

Comments: _____

Physical symptoms after meal: ○ **low** ○ **intense** ○ **non-existent**
○ Belching   ○ Upper abdominal pain and discomfort
○ Nausea   ○ Difficulty or pain with swallowing
○ Stomach fullness or bloating ○ Wheezing or dry cough

Other symptoms: _____

Post-breakfast energy level: ○ low ○ medium ○ high

Lunch   Time: _____

List the foods you ate for lunch.

_____   _____

_____   _____

_____   _____

Drink _____   **Drink** _____
○ room-temp ○ hot ○ cold   ○ room-temp ○ hot ○ cold

Comments: _____

Physical symptoms after meal: ○ **low** ○ **intense** ○ **non-existent**
○ Belching   ○ Upper abdominal pain and discomfort
○ Nausea   ○ Difficulty or pain with swallowing
○ Stomach fullness or bloating ○ Wheezing or dry cough

Other symptoms: _____

Post-lunch energy level: ○ low ○ medium ○ high

Dinner

Time: _____

List the foods you ate for dinner.

_____   _____

_____   _____

_____   _____

Drink _____   **Drink** _____
○ room-temp ○ hot ○ cold   ○ room-temp ○ hot ○ cold

Comments: _____

Physical symptoms after meal: ○ **low**   ○ **intense**   ○ **non-existent**
○ Belching   ○ Upper abdominal pain and discomfort
○ Nausea   ○ Difficulty or pain with swallowing
○ Stomach fullness or bloating   ○ Wheezing or dry cough

Other symptoms: _____

Post-dinner energy level: ○ low   ○ medium   ○ high

Snack

Time: _____

List the foods you ate as a snack.

_____   _____

Drink _____   ○ room-temp   ○ hot   ○ cold

Comments: _____

Post-snack energy level: ○ low   ○ medium   ○ high

Snack

Time: _____

List the foods you ate as a snack.

_____   _____

Drink _____   ○ room-temp   ○ hot   ○ cold

Comments: _____

Post-snack energy level: ○ low   ○ medium   ○ high

Medications & Supplements

Include prescription medication, over-the-counter medication & vitamin supplements.

_____   _____

_____   _____

_____   _____

_____   _____

_____   _____

Energy level | Restfulness

Today's waking energy level?
○ low   ○ medium   ○ high

# of times roused from sleep last night?
○ 1   ○ 2   ○ 3+

Last night's reflux/GERD symptoms:

_____   _____

_____   _____

Bed raised?   ○ Y   ○ N   Wedged Pillows?   ○ Y   ○ N

Last meal time? _____   Approx bedtime? _____   am   pm
(Remember to give yourself at least 2-3 hours after meals before lying down.)

End-of-day notes

Noticeable change in symptoms? _(Ex: "Throat discomfort has completely disappeared.")_

_____

_____

New terms to research   Books & websites with helpful info

_____   _____

_____   _____

Additional notes:

_____

_____

Breakfast

Time: _____

List the foods you ate for breakfast.

_____   _____

_____   _____

_____   _____

Drink _____   **Drink** _____
○ room-temp ○ hot ○ cold   ○ room-temp ○ hot ○ cold

Comments: _____

Physical symptoms after meal: ○ **low** ○ **intense** ○ **non-existent**
○ Belching   ○ Upper abdominal pain and discomfort
○ Nausea   ○ Difficulty or pain with swallowing
○ Stomach fullness or bloating   ○ Wheezing or dry cough

Other symptoms: _____

Post-breakfast energy level: ○ low   ○ medium   ○ high

Lunch

Time: _____

List the foods you ate for lunch.

_____   _____

_____   _____

_____   _____

Drink _____   **Drink** _____
○ room-temp ○ hot ○ cold   ○ room-temp ○ hot ○ cold

Comments: _____

Physical symptoms after meal: ○ **low** ○ **intense** ○ **non-existent**
○ Belching   ○ Upper abdominal pain and discomfort
○ Nausea   ○ Difficulty or pain with swallowing
○ Stomach fullness or bloating   ○ Wheezing or dry cough

Other symptoms: _____

Post-lunch energy level: ○ low   ○ medium   ○ high

Dinner

Time: _____

List the foods you ate for dinner.

_____   _____

_____   _____

_____   _____

Drink _____   **Drink** _____
  ○ room-temp ○ hot ○ cold   ○ room-temp ○ hot ○ cold

Comments: _____

Physical symptoms after meal: ○ **low**   ○ **intense**   ○ **non-existent**
○ Belching   ○ Upper abdominal pain and discomfort
○ Nausea   ○ Difficulty or pain with swallowing
○ Stomach fullness or bloating ○ Wheezing or dry cough

Other symptoms: _____

Post-dinner energy level: ○ low ○ medium ○ high

Snack

Time: _____

List the foods you ate as a snack.

_____   _____

Drink _____   ○ room-temp ○ hot ○ cold

Comments: _____

Post-snack energy level: ○ low ○ medium ○ high

Snack

Time: _____

List the foods you ate as a snack.

_____   _____

Drink _____   ○ room-temp ○ hot ○ cold

Comments: _____

Post-snack energy level: ○ low ○ medium ○ high

Medications & Supplements

Include prescription medication, over-the-counter medication & vitamin supplements.

_____   _____

_____   _____

_____   _____

_____   _____

_____   _____

Energy level | Restfulness

Today's waking energy level?
○ low   ○ medium   ○ high

# of times roused from sleep last night?
○ 1   ○ 2   ○ 3+

Last night's reflux/GERD symptoms:

_____   _____

_____   _____

Bed raised?   ○ Y   ○ N   Wedged Pillows?   ○ Y   ○ N

Last meal time? _____   Approx bedtime? _____ am pm
(Remember to give yourself at least 2-3 hours after meals before lying down.)

End-of-day notes

Noticeable change in symptoms? _(Ex: "Throat discomfort has completely disappeared.")_

_____

_____

New terms to research   Books & websites with helpful info

_____   _____

_____   _____

Additional notes:

_____

_____

Breakfast   Time: _____

List the foods you ate for breakfast.

_____   _____

_____   _____

_____   _____

Drink _____   **Drink** _____
○ room-temp ○ hot ○ cold   ○ room-temp ○ hot ○ cold

Comments: _____

Physical symptoms after meal: ○ **low**   ○ **intense**   ○ **non-existent**
○ Belching   ○ Upper abdominal pain and discomfort
○ Nausea   ○ Difficulty or pain with swallowing
○ Stomach fullness or bloating   ○ Wheezing or dry cough

Other symptoms: _____

Post-breakfast energy level: ○ low ○ medium ○ high

Lunch   Time: _____

List the foods you ate for lunch.

_____   _____

_____   _____

_____   _____

Drink _____   **Drink** _____
○ room-temp ○ hot ○ cold   ○ room-temp ○ hot ○ cold

Comments: _____

Physical symptoms after meal: ○ **low**   ○ **intense**   ○ **non-existent**
○ Belching   ○ Upper abdominal pain and discomfort
○ Nausea   ○ Difficulty or pain with swallowing
○ Stomach fullness or bloating   ○ Wheezing or dry cough

Other symptoms: _____

Post-lunch energy level: ○ low ○ medium ○ high

Dinner

Time: _____

List the foods you ate for dinner.

_____   _____

_____   _____

_____   _____

Drink _____   **Drink** _____
○ room-temp ○ hot ○ cold   ○ room-temp ○ hot ○ cold

Comments:

Physical symptoms after meal: ○ **low** ○ **intense** ○ **non-existent**
○ Belching   ○ Upper abdominal pain and discomfort
○ Nausea   ○ Difficulty or pain with swallowing
○ Stomach fullness or bloating   ○ Wheezing or dry cough

Other symptoms:

Post-dinner energy level: ○ low ○ medium ○ high

Snack

Time: _____

List the foods you ate as a snack.

_____   _____

Drink _____   ○ room-temp ○ hot ○ cold

Comments:

Post-snack energy level: ○ low ○ medium ○ high

Snack

Time: _____

List the foods you ate as a snack.

_____   _____

Drink _____   ○ room-temp ○ hot ○ cold

Comments:

Post-snack energy level: ○ low ○ medium ○ high

Medications & Supplements

Include prescription medication, over-the-counter medication & vitamin supplements.

_____   _____

_____   _____

_____   _____

_____   _____

_____   _____

Energy level | Restfulness

Today's waking energy level?
○ low   ○ medium   ○ high

# of times roused from sleep last night?
○ 1   ○ 2   ○ 3+

Last night's reflux/GERD symptoms:

_____   _____

_____   _____

Bed raised?   ○ Y   ○ N   Wedged Pillows?   ○ Y   ○ N

Last meal time? _____   Approx bedtime? _____   am   pm
(Remember to give yourself at least 2-3 hours after meals before lying down.)

End-of-day notes

Noticeable change in symptoms? *(Ex: "Throat discomfort has completely disappeared.")*

_____

_____

New terms to research   Books & websites with helpful info

_____   _____

_____   _____

Additional notes:

_____

_____

_____

Breakfast

Time: _____

List the foods you ate for breakfast.

_____   _____

_____   _____

_____   _____

Drink _____   **Drink** _____
○ room-temp ○ hot ○ cold   ○ room-temp ○ hot ○ cold

Comments: _____

Physical symptoms after meal: ○ **low**   ○ **intense**   ○ **non-existent**

○ Belching   ○ Upper abdominal pain and discomfort
○ Nausea   ○ Difficulty or pain with swallowing
○ Stomach fullness or bloating   ○ Wheezing or dry cough

Other symptoms: _____

Post-breakfast energy level: ○ low   ○ medium   ○ high

Lunch

Time: _____

List the foods you ate for lunch.

_____   _____

_____   _____

_____   _____

Drink _____   **Drink** _____
○ room-temp ○ hot ○ cold   ○ room-temp ○ hot ○ cold

Comments: _____

Physical symptoms after meal: ○ **low**   ○ **intense**   ○ **non-existent**

○ Belching   ○ Upper abdominal pain and discomfort
○ Nausea   ○ Difficulty or pain with swallowing
○ Stomach fullness or bloating   ○ Wheezing or dry cough

Other symptoms: _____

Post-lunch energy level: ○ low   ○ medium   ○ high

Dinner

Time: _____

List the foods you ate for dinner.

_____   _____

_____   _____

_____   _____

Drink _____   **Drink** _____
○ room-temp   ○ hot   ○ cold   ○ room-temp   ○ hot   ○ cold

Comments: _____

Physical symptoms after meal: ○ **low**   ○ **intense**   ○ **non-existent**
○ Belching   ○ Upper abdominal pain and discomfort
○ Nausea   ○ Difficulty or pain with swallowing
○ Stomach fullness or bloating   ○ Wheezing or dry cough

Other symptoms: _____

Post-dinner energy level: ○ low   ○ medium   ○ high

Snack

Time: _____

List the foods you ate as a snack.

_____   _____

Drink _____   ○ room-temp   ○ hot   ○ cold

Comments: _____

Post-snack energy level: ○ low   ○ medium   ○ high

Snack

Time: _____

List the foods you ate as a snack.

_____   _____

Drink _____   ○ room-temp   ○ hot   ○ cold

Comments: _____

Post-snack energy level: ○ low   ○ medium   ○ high

Medications & Supplements

Include prescription medication, over-the-counter medication & vitamin supplements.

_____   _____

_____   _____

_____   _____

_____   _____

_____   _____

Energy level | Restfulness

Today's waking energy level?
○ low   ○ medium   ○ high

# of times roused from sleep last night?
○ 1   ○ 2   ○ 3+

Last night's reflux/GERD symptoms:

_____   _____

_____   _____

Bed raised?   ○ Y   ○ N   Wedged Pillows?   ○ Y   ○ N

Last meal time? _____   Approx bedtime? _____ am pm
(Remember to give yourself at least 2-3 hours after meals before lying down.)

End-of-day notes

Noticeable change in symptoms? _(Ex: "Throat discomfort has completely disappeared.")_

_____

_____

New terms to research   Books & websites with helpful info

_____   _____

_____   _____

Additional notes:

_____

_____

_____

Breakfast

Time: _____

List the foods you ate for breakfast.

_____   _____

_____   _____

_____   _____

Drink _____   **Drink** _____
  ○ room-temp ○ hot ○ cold   ○ room-temp ○ hot ○ cold

Comments:

Physical symptoms after meal: ○ **low**   ○ **intense**   ○ **non-existent**
○ Belching   ○ Upper abdominal pain and discomfort
○ Nausea   ○ Difficulty or pain with swallowing
○ Stomach fullness or bloating   ○ Wheezing or dry cough

Other symptoms:

Post-breakfast energy level: ○ low ○ medium ○ high

Lunch

Time: _____

List the foods you ate for lunch.

_____   _____

_____   _____

_____   _____

Drink _____   **Drink** _____
  ○ room-temp ○ hot ○ cold   ○ room-temp ○ hot ○ cold

Comments:

Physical symptoms after meal: ○ **low**   ○ **intense**   ○ **non-existent**
○ Belching   ○ Upper abdominal pain and discomfort
○ Nausea   ○ Difficulty or pain with swallowing
○ Stomach fullness or bloating   ○ Wheezing or dry cough

Other symptoms:

Post-lunch energy level: ○ low ○ medium ○ high

Dinner

Time: _____

List the foods you ate for dinner.

_____   _____

_____   _____

_____   _____

Drink _____   **Drink** _____
○ room-temp ○ hot ○ cold   ○ room-temp ○ hot ○ cold

Comments: _____

Physical symptoms after meal: ○ **low** ○ **intense** ○ **non-existent**
○ Belching   ○ Upper abdominal pain and discomfort
○ Nausea   ○ Difficulty or pain with swallowing
○ Stomach fullness or bloating ○ Wheezing or dry cough

Other symptoms: _____

Post-dinner energy level: ○ low ○ medium ○ high

Snack

Time: _____

List the foods you ate as a snack.

_____   _____

Drink _____   ○ room-temp ○ hot ○ cold

Comments: _____

Post-snack energy level: ○ low ○ medium ○ high

Snack

Time: _____

List the foods you ate as a snack.

_____   _____

Drink _____   ○ room-temp ○ hot ○ cold

Comments: _____

Post-snack energy level: ○ low ○ medium ○ high

Medications & Supplements

Include prescription medication, over-the-counter medication & vitamin supplements.

_____   _____

_____   _____

_____   _____

_____   _____

_____   _____

Energy level | Restfulness

Today's waking energy level?
○ low   ○ medium   ○ high

# of times roused from sleep last night?
○ 1   ○ 2   ○ 3+

Last night's reflux/GERD symptoms:

_____   _____

_____   _____

Bed raised?   ○ Y   ○ N   Wedged Pillows?   ○ Y   ○ N

Last meal time? _____   Approx bedtime? _____ am pm
(Remember to give yourself at least 2-3 hours after meals before lying down.)

End-of-day notes

Noticeable change in symptoms? _(Ex: "Throat discomfort has completely disappeared.")_

_____

_____

New terms to research   Books & websites with helpful info

_____   _____

_____   _____

Additional notes:

_____

_____

_____

Breakfast   Time: _____

List the foods you ate for breakfast.

_____   _____

_____   _____

_____   _____

Drink _____   **Drink** _____
   ○ room-temp ○ hot ○ cold   ○ room-temp ○ hot ○ cold

Comments:

Physical symptoms after meal: ○ **low**   ○ **intense**   ○ **non-existent**
○ Belching   ○ Upper abdominal pain and discomfort
○ Nausea   ○ Difficulty or pain with swallowing
○ Stomach fullness or bloating   ○ Wheezing or dry cough

Other symptoms:

Post-breakfast energy level: ○ low ○ medium ○ high

Lunch   Time: _____

List the foods you ate for lunch.

_____   _____

_____   _____

_____   _____

Drink _____   **Drink** _____
   ○ room-temp ○ hot ○ cold   ○ room-temp ○ hot ○ cold

Comments:

Physical symptoms after meal: ○ **low**   ○ **intense**   ○ **non-existent**
○ Belching   ○ Upper abdominal pain and discomfort
○ Nausea   ○ Difficulty or pain with swallowing
○ Stomach fullness or bloating   ○ Wheezing or dry cough

Other symptoms:

Post-lunch energy level: ○ low ○ medium ○ high

Dinner

Time: _____

List the foods you ate for dinner.

_____   _____

_____   _____

_____   _____

Drink _____   **Drink** _____
○ room-temp ○ hot ○ cold   ○ room-temp ○ hot ○ cold

Comments: _____

Physical symptoms after meal: ○ **low**   ○ **intense**   ○ **non-existent**
○ Belching   ○ Upper abdominal pain and discomfort
○ Nausea   ○ Difficulty or pain with swallowing
○ Stomach fullness or bloating   ○ Wheezing or dry cough

Other symptoms: _____

Post-dinner energy level: ○ low   ○ medium   ○ high

Snack

Time: _____

List the foods you ate as a snack.

_____   _____

Drink _____   ○ room-temp ○ hot ○ cold

Comments: _____

Post-snack energy level: ○ low   ○ medium   ○ high

Snack

Time: _____

List the foods you ate as a snack.

_____   _____

Drink _____   ○ room-temp ○ hot ○ cold

Comments: _____

Post-snack energy level: ○ low   ○ medium   ○ high

Medications & Supplements

Include prescription medication, over-the-counter medication & vitamin supplements.

_____   _____

_____   _____

_____   _____

_____   _____

_____   _____

Energy level | Restfulness

Today's waking energy level?
○ low   ○ medium   ○ high

# of times roused from sleep last night?
○ 1   ○ 2   ○ 3+

Last night's reflux/GERD symptoms:

_____   _____

_____   _____

Bed raised?   ○ Y   ○ N   Wedged Pillows?   ○ Y   ○ N

Last meal time? _____   Approx bedtime? _____ am pm
(Remember to give yourself at least 2-3 hours after meals before lying down.)

End-of-day notes

Noticeable change in symptoms? _(Ex: "Throat discomfort has completely disappeared.")_

_____

_____

New terms to research   Books & websites with helpful info

_____   _____

_____   _____

Additional notes:

_____

_____

_____

Breakfast   Time: _____

List the foods you ate for breakfast.

_____   _____

_____   _____

_____   _____

Drink _____   **Drink** _____
   ○ room-temp   ○ hot   ○ cold   ○ room-temp   ○ hot   ○ cold

Comments:

Physical symptoms after meal: ○ **low**   ○ **intense**   ○ **non-existent**
○ Belching   ○ Upper abdominal pain and discomfort
○ Nausea   ○ Difficulty or pain with swallowing
○ Stomach fullness or bloating   ○ Wheezing or dry cough

Other symptoms:

Post-breakfast energy level: ○ low   ○ medium   ○ high

Lunch   Time: _____

List the foods you ate for lunch.

_____   _____

_____   _____

_____   _____

Drink _____   **Drink** _____
   ○ room-temp   ○ hot   ○ cold   ○ room-temp   ○ hot   ○ cold

Comments:

Physical symptoms after meal: ○ **low**   ○ **intense**   ○ **non-existent**
○ Belching   ○ Upper abdominal pain and discomfort
○ Nausea   ○ Difficulty or pain with swallowing
○ Stomach fullness or bloating   ○ Wheezing or dry cough

Other symptoms:

Post-lunch energy level: ○ low   ○ medium   ○ high

Dinner

Time: _____

List the foods you ate for dinner.

_____   _____

_____   _____

_____   _____

Drink _____   **Drink** _____

○ room-temp   ○ hot   ○ cold   ○ room-temp   ○ hot   ○ cold

Comments: _____

Physical symptoms after meal: ○ **low**   ○ **intense**   ○ **non-existent**

○ Belching   ○ Upper abdominal pain and discomfort
○ Nausea   ○ Difficulty or pain with swallowing
○ Stomach fullness or bloating ○ Wheezing or dry cough

Other symptoms: _____

Post-dinner energy level: ○ low   ○ medium   ○ high

Snack

Time: _____

List the foods you ate as a snack.

_____   _____

Drink _____   ○ room-temp   ○ hot   ○ cold

Comments: _____

Post-snack energy level: ○ low   ○ medium   ○ high

Snack

Time: _____

List the foods you ate as a snack.

_____   _____

Drink _____   ○ room-temp   ○ hot   ○ cold

Comments: _____

Post-snack energy level: ○ low   ○ medium   ○ high

Medications & Supplements

Include prescription medication, over-the-counter medication & vitamin supplements.

_____   _____

_____   _____

_____   _____

_____   _____

_____   _____

Energy level | Restfulness

Today's waking energy level?
○ low   ○ medium   ○ high

# of times roused from sleep last night?
○ 1   ○ 2   ○ 3+

Last night's reflux/GERD symptoms:

_____   _____

_____   _____

Bed raised?   ○ Y   ○ N   Wedged Pillows?   ○ Y   ○ N

Last meal time? _____   Approx bedtime? _____ am pm

(Remember to give yourself at least 2-3 hours after meals before lying down.)

End-of-day notes

Noticeable change in symptoms? *(Ex: "Throat discomfort has completely disappeared.")*

_____

_____

New terms to research   Books & websites with helpful info

_____   _____

_____   _____

Additional notes:

_____

_____

_____

Breakfast

Time: _____

List the foods you ate for breakfast.

_____   _____

_____   _____

_____   _____

Drink _____   **Drink** _____
○ room-temp   ○ hot   ○ cold   ○ room-temp   ○ hot   ○ cold

Comments:

Physical symptoms after meal: ○ **low**   ○ **intense**   ○ **non-existent**
○ Belching   ○ Upper abdominal pain and discomfort
○ Nausea   ○ Difficulty or pain with swallowing
○ Stomach fullness or bloating   ○ Wheezing or dry cough

Other symptoms:

Post-breakfast energy level: ○ low   ○ medium   ○ high

Lunch

Time: _____

List the foods you ate for lunch.

_____   _____

_____   _____

_____   _____

Drink _____   **Drink** _____
○ room-temp   ○ hot   ○ cold   ○ room-temp   ○ hot   ○ cold

Comments:

Physical symptoms after meal: ○ **low**   ○ **intense**   ○ **non-existent**
○ Belching   ○ Upper abdominal pain and discomfort
○ Nausea   ○ Difficulty or pain with swallowing
○ Stomach fullness or bloating   ○ Wheezing or dry cough

Other symptoms:

Post-lunch energy level: ○ low   ○ medium   ○ high

Dinner

Time: _____

List the foods you ate for dinner.

_____   _____

_____   _____

_____   _____

Drink _____   **Drink** _____
○ room-temp ○ hot ○ cold   ○ room-temp ○ hot ○ cold

Comments: _____

Physical symptoms after meal: ○ **low**   ○ **intense**   ○ **non-existent**
○ Belching   ○ Upper abdominal pain and discomfort
○ Nausea   ○ Difficulty or pain with swallowing
○ Stomach fullness or bloating   ○ Wheezing or dry cough

Other symptoms: _____

Post-dinner energy level: ○ low   ○ medium   ○ high

Snack

Time: _____

List the foods you ate as a snack.

_____   _____

Drink _____   ○ room-temp ○ hot ○ cold

Comments: _____

Post-snack energy level: ○ low   ○ medium   ○ high

Snack

Time: _____

List the foods you ate as a snack.

_____   _____

Drink _____   ○ room-temp ○ hot ○ cold

Comments: _____

Post-snack energy level: ○ low   ○ medium   ○ high

Medications & Supplements

Include prescription medication, over-the-counter medication & vitamin supplements.

_____   _____

_____   _____

_____   _____

_____   _____

_____   _____

Energy level | Restfulness

Today's waking energy level?
○ low   ○ medium   ○ high

# of times roused from sleep last night?
○ 1   ○ 2   ○ 3+

Last night's reflux/GERD symptoms:

_____   _____

_____   _____

Bed raised?   ○ Y   ○ N   Wedged Pillows?   ○ Y   ○ N

Last meal time? _____   Approx bedtime? _____ am pm
(Remember to give yourself at least 2-3 hours after meals before lying down.)

End-of-day notes

Noticeable change in symptoms? *(Ex: "Throat discomfort has completely disappeared.")*

_____

_____

New terms to research   Books & websites with helpful info

_____   _____

_____   _____

Additional notes:

_____

_____

_____

Breakfast   Time: _____

List the foods you ate for breakfast.

_____   _____

_____   _____

_____   _____

Drink _____   **Drink** _____
  ○ room-temp ○ hot ○ cold   ○ room-temp ○ hot ○ cold

Comments:

Physical symptoms after meal: ○ **low**   ○ **intense**   ○ **non-existent**
○ Belching   ○ Upper abdominal pain and discomfort
○ Nausea   ○ Difficulty or pain with swallowing
○ Stomach fullness or bloating   ○ Wheezing or dry cough

Other symptoms:

Post-breakfast energy level: ○ low ○ medium ○ high

Lunch   Time: _____

List the foods you ate for lunch.

_____   _____

_____   _____

_____   _____

Drink _____   **Drink** _____
  ○ room-temp ○ hot ○ cold   ○ room-temp ○ hot ○ cold

Comments:

Physical symptoms after meal: ○ **low**   ○ **intense**   ○ **non-existent**
○ Belching   ○ Upper abdominal pain and discomfort
○ Nausea   ○ Difficulty or pain with swallowing
○ Stomach fullness or bloating   ○ Wheezing or dry cough

Other symptoms:

Post-lunch energy level: ○ low ○ medium ○ high

Dinner

Time: _____

List the foods you ate for dinner.

_____   _____

_____   _____

_____   _____

Drink _____   **Drink** _____
  ○ room-temp ○ hot ○ cold   ○ room-temp ○ hot ○ cold

Comments: _____

Physical symptoms after meal: ○ **low** ○ **intense** ○ **non-existent**
- ○ Belching
- ○ Nausea
- ○ Stomach fullness or bloating
- ○ Upper abdominal pain and discomfort
- ○ Difficulty or pain with swallowing
- ○ Wheezing or dry cough

Other symptoms: _____

Post-dinner energy level: ○ low ○ medium ○ high

Snack

Time: _____

List the foods you ate as a snack.

_____   _____

Drink _____ ○ room-temp ○ hot ○ cold

Comments: _____

Post-snack energy level: ○ low ○ medium ○ high

Snack

Time: _____

List the foods you ate as a snack.

_____   _____

Drink _____ ○ room-temp ○ hot ○ cold

Comments: _____

Post-snack energy level: ○ low ○ medium ○ high

Medications & Supplements

Include prescription medication, over-the-counter medication & vitamin supplements.

_____   _____

_____   _____

_____   _____

_____   _____

_____   _____

Energy level | Restfulness

Today's waking energy level?
○ low   ○ medium   ○ high

# of times roused from sleep last night?
○ 1   ○ 2   ○ 3+

Last night's reflux/GERD symptoms:

_____   _____

_____   _____

Bed raised?   ○ Y   ○ N   Wedged Pillows?   ○ Y   ○ N

Last meal time? _____   Approx bedtime? _____ am pm
(Remember to give yourself at least 2-3 hours after meals before lying down.)

End-of-day notes

Noticeable change in symptoms? _(Ex: "Throat discomfort has completely disappeared.")_

_____

_____

New terms to research   Books & websites with helpful info

_____   _____

_____   _____

Additional notes:

_____

_____

_____

_____

Breakfast

Time: _____

List the foods you ate for breakfast.

_____   _____

_____   _____

_____   _____

Drink _____   **Drink** _____
○ room-temp   ○ hot   ○ cold   ○ room-temp   ○ hot   ○ cold

Comments: _____

Physical symptoms after meal: ○ **low**   ○ **intense**   ○ **non-existent**
○ Belching   ○ Upper abdominal pain and discomfort
○ Nausea   ○ Difficulty or pain with swallowing
○ Stomach fullness or bloating   ○ Wheezing or dry cough

Other symptoms: _____

Post-breakfast energy level: ○ low   ○ medium   ○ high

Lunch

Time: _____

List the foods you ate for lunch.

_____   _____

_____   _____

_____   _____

Drink _____   **Drink** _____
○ room-temp   ○ hot   ○ cold   ○ room-temp   ○ hot   ○ cold

Comments: _____

Physical symptoms after meal: ○ **low**   ○ **intense**   ○ **non-existent**
○ Belching   ○ Upper abdominal pain and discomfort
○ Nausea   ○ Difficulty or pain with swallowing
○ Stomach fullness or bloating   ○ Wheezing or dry cough

Other symptoms: _____

Post-lunch energy level: ○ low   ○ medium   ○ high

Dinner

Time: _____

List the foods you ate for dinner.

_____   _____

_____   _____

_____   _____

Drink _____   **Drink** _____
○ room-temp ○ hot ○ cold   ○ room-temp ○ hot ○ cold

Comments:

Physical symptoms after meal: ○ **low**   ○ **intense**   ○ **non-existent**
○ Belching   ○ Upper abdominal pain and discomfort
○ Nausea   ○ Difficulty or pain with swallowing
○ Stomach fullness or bloating ○ Wheezing or dry cough

Other symptoms:

Post-dinner energy level: ○ low   ○ medium   ○ high

Snack

Time: _____

List the foods you ate as a snack.

_____   _____

Drink _____   ○ room-temp   ○ hot   ○ cold

Comments:

Post-snack energy level: ○ low   ○ medium   ○ high

Snack

Time: _____

List the foods you ate as a snack.

_____   _____

Drink _____   ○ room-temp   ○ hot   ○ cold

Comments:

Post-snack energy level: ○ low   ○ medium   ○ high

Medications & Supplements

Include prescription medication, over-the-counter medication & vitamin supplements.

_____   _____

_____   _____

_____   _____

_____   _____

_____   _____

Energy level | Restfulness

Today's waking energy level?
○ low   ○ medium   ○ high

# of times roused from sleep last night?
○ 1   ○ 2   ○ 3+

Last night's reflux/GERD symptoms:

_____   _____

_____   _____

Bed raised?   ○ Y   ○ N   Wedged Pillows?   ○ Y   ○ N

Last meal time? _____   Approx bedtime? _____ am pm
(Remember to give yourself at least 2-3 hours after meals before lying down.)

End-of-day notes

Noticeable change in symptoms? _(Ex: "Throat discomfort has completely disappeared.")_

_____

_____

New terms to research   Books & websites with helpful info

_____   _____

_____   _____

Additional notes:

_____

_____

_____

Breakfast   Time: _____

List the foods you ate for breakfast.

_____   _____

_____   _____

_____   _____

Drink _____   **Drink** _____
○ room-temp ○ hot ○ cold   ○ room-temp ○ hot ○ cold

Comments: _____

Physical symptoms after meal: ○ **low** ○ **intense** ○ **non-existent**
○ Belching   ○ Upper abdominal pain and discomfort
○ Nausea   ○ Difficulty or pain with swallowing
○ Stomach fullness or bloating ○ Wheezing or dry cough

Other symptoms: _____

Post-breakfast energy level: ○ low ○ medium ○ high

Lunch   Time: _____

List the foods you ate for lunch.

_____   _____

_____   _____

_____   _____

Drink _____   **Drink** _____
○ room-temp ○ hot ○ cold   ○ room-temp ○ hot ○ cold

Comments: _____

Physical symptoms after meal: ○ **low** ○ **intense** ○ **non-existent**
○ Belching   ○ Upper abdominal pain and discomfort
○ Nausea   ○ Difficulty or pain with swallowing
○ Stomach fullness or bloating ○ Wheezing or dry cough

Other symptoms: _____

Post-lunch energy level: ○ low ○ medium ○ high

Dinner

Time: _____

List the foods you ate for dinner.

_____   _____

_____   _____

_____   _____

Drink _____   **Drink** _____
○ room-temp ○ hot ○ cold   ○ room-temp ○ hot ○ cold

Comments: _____

Physical symptoms after meal: ○ **low**   ○ **intense**   ○ **non-existent**
○ Belching   ○ Upper abdominal pain and discomfort
○ Nausea   ○ Difficulty or pain with swallowing
○ Stomach fullness or bloating   ○ Wheezing or dry cough

Other symptoms: _____

Post-dinner energy level: ○ low ○ medium ○ high

Snack

Time: _____

List the foods you ate as a snack.

_____   _____

Drink _____   ○ room-temp ○ hot ○ cold

Comments: _____

Post-snack energy level: ○ low ○ medium ○ high

Snack

Time: _____

List the foods you ate as a snack.

_____   _____

Drink _____   ○ room-temp ○ hot ○ cold

Comments: _____

Post-snack energy level: ○ low ○ medium ○ high

Medications & Supplements

Include prescription medication, over-the-counter medication & vitamin supplements.

_____   _____

_____   _____

_____   _____

_____   _____

_____   _____

Energy level | Restfulness

Today's waking energy level?
○ low   ○ medium   ○ high

# of times roused from sleep last night?
○ 1   ○ 2   ○ 3+

Last night's reflux/GERD symptoms:

_____   _____

_____   _____

Bed raised?   ○ Y   ○ N   Wedged Pillows?   ○ Y   ○ N

Last meal time? _____   Approx bedtime? _____ am pm
(Remember to give yourself at least 2-3 hours after meals before lying down.)

End-of-day notes

Noticeable change in symptoms? _(Ex: "Throat discomfort has completely disappeared.")_

_____

_____

New terms to research   Books & websites with helpful info

_____   _____

_____   _____

Additional notes:

_____

_____

_____

Breakfast

Time: _____

List the foods you ate for breakfast.

_____   _____

_____   _____

_____

Drink _____   **Drink** _____

○ room-temp   ○ hot   ○ cold   ○ room-temp   ○ hot   ○ cold

Comments:

Physical symptoms after meal: ○ **low**   ○ **intense**   ○ **non-existent**

○ Belching   ○ Upper abdominal pain and discomfort

○ Nausea   ○ Difficulty or pain with swallowing

○ Stomach fullness or bloating   ○ Wheezing or dry cough

Other symptoms:

Post-breakfast energy level: ○ low   ○ medium   ○ high

Lunch

Time: _____

List the foods you ate for lunch.

_____   _____

_____   _____

_____

Drink _____   **Drink** _____

○ room-temp   ○ hot   ○ cold   ○ room-temp   ○ hot   ○ cold

Comments:

Physical symptoms after meal: ○ **low**   ○ **intense**   ○ **non-existent**

○ Belching   ○ Upper abdominal pain and discomfort

○ Nausea   ○ Difficulty or pain with swallowing

○ Stomach fullness or bloating   ○ Wheezing or dry cough

Other symptoms:

Post-lunch energy level: ○ low   ○ medium   ○ high

Dinner

Time: _____

List the foods you ate for dinner.

_____   _____

_____   _____

_____   _____

Drink _____   **Drink** _____
○ room-temp   ○ hot   ○ cold   ○ room-temp   ○ hot   ○ cold

Comments: _____

Physical symptoms after meal: ○ **low**   ○ **intense**   ○ **non-existent**
○ Belching   ○ Upper abdominal pain and discomfort
○ Nausea   ○ Difficulty or pain with swallowing
○ Stomach fullness or bloating   ○ Wheezing or dry cough

Other symptoms: _____

Post-dinner energy level: ○ low   ○ medium   ○ high

Snack

Time: _____

List the foods you ate as a snack.

_____   _____

Drink _____   ○ room-temp   ○ hot   ○ cold

Comments: _____

Post-snack energy level: ○ low   ○ medium   ○ high

Snack

Time: _____

List the foods you ate as a snack.

_____   _____

Drink _____   ○ room-temp   ○ hot   ○ cold

Comments: _____

Post-snack energy level: ○ low   ○ medium   ○ high

Medications & Supplements

Include prescription medication, over-the-counter medication & vitamin supplements.

_____   _____

_____   _____

_____   _____

_____   _____

_____   _____

Energy level | Restfulness

Today's waking energy level?
○ low   ○ medium   ○ high

# of times roused from sleep last night?
○ 1   ○ 2   ○ 3+

Last night's reflux/GERD symptoms:

_____   _____

_____   _____

Bed raised?   ○ Y   ○ N   Wedged Pillows?   ○ Y   ○ N

Last meal time? _____   Approx bedtime? _____   am   pm
    (Remember to give yourself at least 2-3 hours after meals before lying down.)

End-of-day notes

Noticeable change in symptoms? _(Ex: "Throat discomfort has completely disappeared.")_

_____

_____

New terms to research   Books & websites with helpful info

_____   _____

_____   _____

Additional notes:

_____

_____

_____

Breakfast   Time: _____

List the foods you ate for breakfast.

_____   _____

_____   _____

_____   _____

Drink _____   **Drink** _____
   o room-temp o hot o cold   o room-temp o hot o cold

Comments:

Physical symptoms after meal: o **low** o **intense** o **non-existent**
o Belching   o Upper abdominal pain and discomfort
o Nausea   o Difficulty or pain with swallowing
o Stomach fullness or bloating o Wheezing or dry cough

Other symptoms:

Post-breakfast energy level: o low o medium o high

Lunch   Time: _____

List the foods you ate for lunch.

_____   _____

_____   _____

_____   _____

Drink _____   **Drink** _____
   o room-temp o hot o cold   o room-temp o hot o cold

Comments:

Physical symptoms after meal: o **low** o **intense** o **non-existent**
o Belching   o Upper abdominal pain and discomfort
o Nausea   o Difficulty or pain with swallowing
o Stomach fullness or bloating o Wheezing or dry cough

Other symptoms:

Post-lunch energy level: o low o medium o high

Dinner

Time: _____

List the foods you ate for dinner.

_____   _____

_____   _____

_____   _____

Drink _____   **Drink** _____
○ room-temp   ○ hot   ○ cold   ○ room-temp   ○ hot   ○ cold

Comments: _____

Physical symptoms after meal: ○ **low**   ○ **intense**   ○ **non-existent**

○ Belching   ○ Upper abdominal pain and discomfort

○ Nausea   ○ Difficulty or pain with swallowing

○ Stomach fullness or bloating   ○ Wheezing or dry cough

Other symptoms: _____

Post-dinner energy level: ○ low   ○ medium   ○ high

Snack

Time: _____

List the foods you ate as a snack.

_____   _____

Drink _____   ○ room-temp   ○ hot   ○ cold

Comments: _____

Post-snack energy level: ○ low   ○ medium   ○ high

Snack

Time: _____

List the foods you ate as a snack.

_____   _____

Drink _____   ○ room-temp   ○ hot   ○ cold

Comments: _____

Post-snack energy level: ○ low   ○ medium   ○ high

Medications & Supplements

Include prescription medication, over-the-counter medication & vitamin supplements.

_____   _____

_____   _____

_____   _____

_____   _____

_____   _____

Energy level | Restfulness

Today's waking energy level?
○ low   ○ medium   ○ high

# of times roused from sleep last night?
○ 1   ○ 2   ○ 3+

Last night's reflux/GERD symptoms:

_____   _____

_____   _____

Bed raised?   ○ Y   ○ N   Wedged Pillows?   ○ Y   ○ N

Last meal time? _____   Approx bedtime? _____ am pm
(Remember to give yourself at least 2-3 hours after meals before lying down.)

End-of-day notes

Noticeable change in symptoms? _(Ex: "Throat discomfort has completely disappeared.")_

_____

_____

New terms to research   Books & websites with helpful info

_____   _____

_____   _____

Additional notes:

_____

_____

_____

Breakfast   Time: _____

List the foods you ate for breakfast.

_____   _____

_____   _____

_____   _____

Drink _____   **Drink** _____
○ room-temp   ○ hot   ○ cold   ○ room-temp   ○ hot   ○ cold

Comments: _____

Physical symptoms after meal: ○ **low**   ○ **intense**   ○ **non-existent**
○ Belching   ○ Upper abdominal pain and discomfort
○ Nausea   ○ Difficulty or pain with swallowing
○ Stomach fullness or bloating   ○ Wheezing or dry cough

Other symptoms: _____

Post-breakfast energy level: ○ low   ○ medium   ○ high

Lunch   Time: _____

List the foods you ate for lunch.

_____   _____

_____   _____

_____   _____

Drink _____   **Drink** _____
○ room-temp   ○ hot   ○ cold   ○ room-temp   ○ hot   ○ cold

Comments: _____

Physical symptoms after meal: ○ **low**   ○ **intense**   ○ **non-existent**
○ Belching   ○ Upper abdominal pain and discomfort
○ Nausea   ○ Difficulty or pain with swallowing
○ Stomach fullness or bloating   ○ Wheezing or dry cough

Other symptoms: _____

Post-lunch energy level: ○ low   ○ medium   ○ high

Dinner

Time: _____

List the foods you ate for dinner.

_____   _____

_____   _____

_____   _____

Drink _____   **Drink** _____
  ○ room-temp ○ hot ○ cold   ○ room-temp ○ hot ○ cold

Comments:
_____

Physical symptoms after meal: ○ **low**   ○ **intense**   ○ **non-existent**
○ Belching   ○ Upper abdominal pain and discomfort
○ Nausea   ○ Difficulty or pain with swallowing
○ Stomach fullness or bloating   ○ Wheezing or dry cough

Other symptoms:
_____

Post-dinner energy level: ○ low   ○ medium   ○ high

Snack

Time: _____

List the foods you ate as a snack.

_____   _____

Drink _____   ○ room-temp   ○ hot   ○ cold

Comments:
_____

Post-snack energy level: ○ low   ○ medium   ○ high

Snack

Time: _____

List the foods you ate as a snack.

_____   _____

Drink _____   ○ room-temp   ○ hot   ○ cold

Comments:
_____

Post-snack energy level: ○ low   ○ medium   ○ high

Medications & Supplements

Include prescription medication, over-the-counter medication & vitamin supplements.

_____   _____

_____   _____

_____   _____

_____   _____

_____   _____

Energy level | Restfulness

Today's waking energy level?
○ low   ○ medium   ○ high

# of times roused from sleep last night?
○ 1   ○ 2   ○ 3+

Last night's reflux/GERD symptoms:

_____   _____

_____   _____

Bed raised?   ○ Y   ○ N   Wedged Pillows?   ○ Y   ○ N

Last meal time? _____   Approx bedtime? _____ am   pm
(Remember to give yourself at least 2-3 hours after meals before lying down.)

End-of-day notes

Noticeable change in symptoms? _(Ex: "Throat discomfort has completely disappeared.")_

_____

_____

New terms to research   Books & websites with helpful info

_____   _____

_____   _____

Additional notes:

_____

_____

_____

Breakfast   Time: _____

List the foods you ate for breakfast.

_____   _____

_____   _____

_____   _____

Drink _____   **Drink** _____
  ○ room-temp ○ hot ○ cold   ○ room-temp ○ hot ○ cold

Comments:

Physical symptoms after meal: ○ **low**   ○ **intense**   ○ **non-existent**
○ Belching   ○ Upper abdominal pain and discomfort
○ Nausea   ○ Difficulty or pain with swallowing
○ Stomach fullness or bloating   ○ Wheezing or dry cough

Other symptoms:

Post-breakfast energy level: ○ low   ○ medium   ○ high

Lunch   Time: _____

List the foods you ate for lunch.

_____   _____

_____   _____

_____   _____

Drink _____   **Drink** _____
  ○ room-temp ○ hot ○ cold   ○ room-temp ○ hot ○ cold

Comments:

Physical symptoms after meal: ○ **low**   ○ **intense**   ○ **non-existent**
○ Belching   ○ Upper abdominal pain and discomfort
○ Nausea   ○ Difficulty or pain with swallowing
○ Stomach fullness or bloating   ○ Wheezing or dry cough

Other symptoms:

Post-lunch energy level: ○ low   ○ medium   ○ high

Dinner

Time: _____

List the foods you ate for dinner.

_____   _____

_____   _____

_____   _____

Drink _____   **Drink** _____
○ room-temp ○ hot ○ cold   ○ room-temp ○ hot ○ cold

Comments: _____

Physical symptoms after meal: ○ **low** ○ **intense** ○ **non-existent**
○ Belching   ○ Upper abdominal pain and discomfort
○ Nausea   ○ Difficulty or pain with swallowing
○ Stomach fullness or bloating   ○ Wheezing or dry cough

Other symptoms: _____

Post-dinner energy level: ○ low ○ medium ○ high

Snack

Time: _____

List the foods you ate as a snack.

_____   _____

Drink _____ ○ room-temp ○ hot ○ cold

Comments: _____

Post-snack energy level: ○ low ○ medium ○ high

Snack

Time: _____

List the foods you ate as a snack.

_____   _____

Drink _____ ○ room-temp ○ hot ○ cold

Comments: _____

Post-snack energy level: ○ low ○ medium ○ high

Medications & Supplements

Include prescription medication, over-the-counter medication & vitamin supplements.

_____   _____

_____   _____

_____   _____

_____   _____

_____   _____

Energy level | Restfulness

Today's waking energy level?
○ low   ○ medium   ○ high

# of times roused from sleep last night?
○ 1   ○ 2   ○ 3+

Last night's reflux/GERD symptoms:

_____   _____

_____   _____

Bed raised?   ○ Y   ○ N   Wedged Pillows?   ○ Y   ○ N

Last meal time? _____   Approx bedtime? _____ am pm
(Remember to give yourself at least 2-3 hours after meals before lying down.)

End-of-day notes

Noticeable change in symptoms? _(Ex: "Throat discomfort has completely disappeared.")_

_____

_____

New terms to research   Books & websites with helpful info

_____   _____

_____   _____

Additional notes:

_____

_____

_____

Breakfast

Time: _____

List the foods you ate for breakfast.

_____ _____

_____ _____

_____ _____

Drink _____ **Drink** _____
○ room-temp ○ hot ○ cold   ○ room-temp ○ hot ○ cold

Comments: _____

Physical symptoms after meal: ○ **low** ○ **intense** ○ **non-existent**
○ Belching   ○ Upper abdominal pain and discomfort
○ Nausea   ○ Difficulty or pain with swallowing
○ Stomach fullness or bloating ○ Wheezing or dry cough

Other symptoms: _____

Post-breakfast energy level: ○ low ○ medium ○ high

Lunch

Time: _____

List the foods you ate for lunch.

_____ _____

_____ _____

_____ _____

Drink _____ **Drink** _____
○ room-temp ○ hot ○ cold   ○ room-temp ○ hot ○ cold

Comments: _____

Physical symptoms after meal: ○ **low** ○ **intense** ○ **non-existent**
○ Belching   ○ Upper abdominal pain and discomfort
○ Nausea   ○ Difficulty or pain with swallowing
○ Stomach fullness or bloating ○ Wheezing or dry cough

Other symptoms: _____

Post-lunch energy level: ○ low ○ medium ○ high

Dinner

Time: _____

List the foods you ate for dinner.

_____   _____

_____   _____

_____   _____

Drink _____   **Drink** _____
○ room-temp ○ hot ○ cold   ○ room-temp ○ hot ○ cold

Comments: _____

Physical symptoms after meal: ○ **low** ○ **intense** ○ **non-existent**
○ Belching   ○ Upper abdominal pain and discomfort
○ Nausea   ○ Difficulty or pain with swallowing
○ Stomach fullness or bloating ○ Wheezing or dry cough

Other symptoms: _____

Post-dinner energy level: ○ low ○ medium ○ high

Snack

Time: _____

List the foods you ate as a snack.

_____   _____

Drink _____   ○ room-temp ○ hot ○ cold

Comments: _____

Post-snack energy level: ○ low ○ medium ○ high

Snack

Time: _____

List the foods you ate as a snack.

_____   _____

Drink _____   ○ room-temp ○ hot ○ cold

Comments: _____

Post-snack energy level: ○ low ○ medium ○ high

Medications & Supplements

Include prescription medication, over-the-counter medication & vitamin supplements.

_____   _____

_____   _____

_____   _____

_____   _____

_____   _____

Energy level | Restfulness

Today's waking energy level?
○ low   ○ medium   ○ high

# of times roused from sleep last night?
○ 1   ○ 2   ○ 3+

Last night's reflux/GERD symptoms:

_____   _____

_____   _____

Bed raised?   ○ Y   ○ N   Wedged Pillows?   ○ Y   ○ N

Last meal time? _____   Approx bedtime? _____ am pm
(Remember to give yourself at least 2-3 hours after meals before lying down.)

End-of-day notes

Noticeable change in symptoms? _(Ex: "Throat discomfort has completely disappeared.")_

_____

_____

New terms to research   Books & websites with helpful info

_____   _____

_____   _____

Additional notes:

_____

_____

_____

Breakfast   Time: _____

List the foods you ate for breakfast.

_____   _____

_____   _____

_____   _____

Drink _____   **Drink** _____
○ room-temp   ○ hot   ○ cold   ○ room-temp   ○ hot   ○ cold

Comments:

Physical symptoms after meal: ○ **low**   ○ **intense**   ○ **non-existent**
○ Belching   ○ Upper abdominal pain and discomfort
○ Nausea   ○ Difficulty or pain with swallowing
○ Stomach fullness or bloating   ○ Wheezing or dry cough

Other symptoms:

Post-breakfast energy level: ○ low   ○ medium   ○ high

Lunch   Time: _____

List the foods you ate for lunch.

_____   _____

_____   _____

_____   _____

Drink _____   **Drink** _____
○ room-temp   ○ hot   ○ cold   ○ room-temp   ○ hot   ○ cold

Comments:

Physical symptoms after meal: ○ **low**   ○ **intense**   ○ **non-existent**
○ Belching   ○ Upper abdominal pain and discomfort
○ Nausea   ○ Difficulty or pain with swallowing
○ Stomach fullness or bloating   ○ Wheezing or dry cough

Other symptoms:

Post-lunch energy level: ○ low   ○ medium   ○ high

Dinner

Time: _____

List the foods you ate for dinner.

_____   _____

_____   _____

_____   _____

Drink _____   **Drink** _____
○ room-temp ○ hot ○ cold   ○ room-temp ○ hot ○ cold

Comments: _____

Physical symptoms after meal: ○ **low**   ○ **intense**   ○ **non-existent**
○ Belching   ○ Upper abdominal pain and discomfort
○ Nausea   ○ Difficulty or pain with swallowing
○ Stomach fullness or bloating   ○ Wheezing or dry cough

Other symptoms: _____

Post-dinner energy level: ○ low   ○ medium   ○ high

Snack

Time: _____

List the foods you ate as a snack.

_____   _____

Drink _____   ○ room-temp ○ hot ○ cold

Comments: _____

Post-snack energy level: ○ low   ○ medium   ○ high

Snack

Time: _____

List the foods you ate as a snack.

_____   _____

Drink _____   ○ room-temp ○ hot ○ cold

Comments: _____

Post-snack energy level: ○ low   ○ medium   ○ high

Medications & Supplements

Include prescription medication, over-the-counter medication & vitamin supplements.

_____   _____

_____   _____

_____   _____

_____   _____

_____   _____

Energy level | Restfulness

Today's waking energy level?
○ low   ○ medium   ○ high

# of times roused from sleep last night?
○ 1   ○ 2   ○ 3+

Last night's reflux/GERD symptoms:

_____   _____

_____   _____

Bed raised?   ○ Y   ○ N   Wedged Pillows?   ○ Y   ○ N

Last meal time? _____   Approx bedtime? _____ am pm
(Remember to give yourself at least 2-3 hours after meals before lying down.)

End-of-day notes

Noticeable change in symptoms? _(Ex: "Throat discomfort has completely disappeared.")_

_____

_____

New terms to research   Books & websites with helpful info

_____   _____

_____   _____

Additional notes:

_____

_____

_____

Breakfast   Time: _____

List the foods you ate for breakfast.

_____   _____

_____   _____

_____   _____

Drink _____   **Drink** _____
  ○ room-temp ○ hot ○ cold   ○ room-temp ○ hot ○ cold

Comments: _____

Physical symptoms after meal: ○ **low**   ○ **intense**   ○ **non-existent**
- ○ Belching
- ○ Nausea
- ○ Stomach fullness or bloating
- ○ Upper abdominal pain and discomfort
- ○ Difficulty or pain with swallowing
- ○ Wheezing or dry cough

Other symptoms: _____

Post-breakfast energy level: ○ low   ○ medium   ○ high

Lunch   Time: _____

List the foods you ate for lunch.

_____   _____

_____   _____

_____   _____

Drink _____   **Drink** _____
  ○ room-temp ○ hot ○ cold   ○ room-temp ○ hot ○ cold

Comments: _____

Physical symptoms after meal: ○ **low**   ○ **intense**   ○ **non-existent**
- ○ Belching
- ○ Nausea
- ○ Stomach fullness or bloating
- ○ Upper abdominal pain and discomfort
- ○ Difficulty or pain with swallowing
- ○ Wheezing or dry cough

Other symptoms: _____

Post-lunch energy level: ○ low   ○ medium   ○ high

Dinner

Time: _____

List the foods you ate for dinner.

_____   _____

_____   _____

_____   _____

Drink _____   **Drink** _____
 ○ room-temp ○ hot ○ cold   ○ room-temp ○ hot ○ cold

Comments: _____

Physical symptoms after meal: ○ **low** ○ **intense** ○ **non-existent**
 ○ Belching   ○ Upper abdominal pain and discomfort
 ○ Nausea   ○ Difficulty or pain with swallowing
 ○ Stomach fullness or bloating   ○ Wheezing or dry cough

Other symptoms: _____

Post-dinner energy level: ○ low ○ medium ○ high

Snack

Time: _____

List the foods you ate as a snack.

_____   _____

Drink _____   ○ room-temp ○ hot ○ cold

Comments: _____

Post-snack energy level: ○ low ○ medium ○ high

Snack

Time: _____

List the foods you ate as a snack.

_____   _____

Drink _____   ○ room-temp ○ hot ○ cold

Comments: _____

Post-snack energy level: ○ low ○ medium ○ high

Medications & Supplements

Include prescription medication, over-the-counter medication & vitamin supplements.

_____   _____

_____   _____

_____   _____

_____   _____

_____   _____

Energy level | Restfulness

Today's waking energy level?
○ low   ○ medium   ○ high

# of times roused from sleep last night?
○ 1   ○ 2   ○ 3+

Last night's reflux/GERD symptoms:

_____   _____

_____   _____

Bed raised?   ○ Y   ○ N   Wedged Pillows?   ○ Y   ○ N

Last meal time? _____   Approx bedtime? _____ am pm
(Remember to give yourself at least 2-3 hours after meals before lying down.)

End-of-day notes

Noticeable change in symptoms? _(Ex: "Throat discomfort has completely disappeared.")_

_____

_____

New terms to research   Books & websites with helpful info

_____   _____

_____   _____

Additional notes:

_____

_____

_____

Breakfast

Time: _____

List the foods you ate for breakfast.

_____   _____

_____   _____

_____   _____

Drink _____   **Drink** _____
○ room-temp ○ hot ○ cold   ○ room-temp ○ hot ○ cold

Comments:

Physical symptoms after meal: ○ **low**   ○ **intense**   ○ **non-existent**
○ Belching   ○ Upper abdominal pain and discomfort
○ Nausea   ○ Difficulty or pain with swallowing
○ Stomach fullness or bloating   ○ Wheezing or dry cough

Other symptoms:

Post-breakfast energy level: ○ low   ○ medium   ○ high

Lunch

Time: _____

List the foods you ate for lunch.

_____   _____

_____   _____

_____   _____

Drink _____   **Drink** _____
○ room-temp ○ hot ○ cold   ○ room-temp ○ hot ○ cold

Comments:

Physical symptoms after meal: ○ **low**   ○ **intense**   ○ **non-existent**
○ Belching   ○ Upper abdominal pain and discomfort
○ Nausea   ○ Difficulty or pain with swallowing
○ Stomach fullness or bloating   ○ Wheezing or dry cough

Other symptoms:

Post-lunch energy level: ○ low   ○ medium   ○ high

Dinner

Time: _____

List the foods you ate for dinner.

_____   _____

_____   _____

_____   _____

Drink _____   **Drink** _____
○ room-temp ○ hot ○ cold   ○ room-temp ○ hot ○ cold

Comments:

Physical symptoms after meal: ○ **low**   ○ **intense**   ○ **non-existent**
○ Belching   ○ Upper abdominal pain and discomfort
○ Nausea   ○ Difficulty or pain with swallowing
○ Stomach fullness or bloating   ○ Wheezing or dry cough

Other symptoms:

Post-dinner energy level: ○ low   ○ medium   ○ high

Snack

Time: _____

List the foods you ate as a snack.

_____   _____

Drink _____   ○ room-temp   ○ hot   ○ cold

Comments:

Post-snack energy level: ○ low   ○ medium   ○ high

Snack

Time: _____

List the foods you ate as a snack.

_____   _____

Drink _____   ○ room-temp   ○ hot   ○ cold

Comments:

Post-snack energy level: ○ low   ○ medium   ○ high

Medications & Supplements

Include prescription medication, over-the-counter medication & vitamin supplements.

_____   _____

_____   _____

_____   _____

_____   _____

_____   _____

Energy level | Restfulness

Today's waking energy level?
○ low   ○ medium   ○ high

# of times roused from sleep last night?
○ 1   ○ 2   ○ 3+

Last night's reflux/GERD symptoms:

_____   _____

_____   _____

Bed raised?   ○ Y   ○ N   Wedged Pillows?   ○ Y   ○ N

Last meal time? _____   Approx bedtime? _____ am pm
(Remember to give yourself at least 2-3 hours after meals before lying down.)

End-of-day notes

Noticeable change in symptoms? _(Ex: "Throat discomfort has completely disappeared.")_

_____

_____

New terms to research   Books & websites with helpful info

_____   _____

_____   _____

Additional notes:

_____

_____

_____

Breakfast   Time: _____

List the foods you ate for breakfast.

_____   _____

_____   _____

_____   _____

Drink _____   **Drink** _____
  ○ room-temp ○ hot ○ cold   ○ room-temp ○ hot ○ cold

Comments: _____

Physical symptoms after meal: ○ **low** ○ **intense** ○ **non-existent**
○ Belching   ○ Upper abdominal pain and discomfort
○ Nausea   ○ Difficulty or pain with swallowing
○ Stomach fullness or bloating   ○ Wheezing or dry cough

Other symptoms: _____

Post-breakfast energy level: ○ low ○ medium ○ high

Lunch   Time: _____

List the foods you ate for lunch.

_____   _____

_____   _____

_____   _____

Drink _____   **Drink** _____
  ○ room-temp ○ hot ○ cold   ○ room-temp ○ hot ○ cold

Comments: _____

Physical symptoms after meal: ○ **low** ○ **intense** ○ **non-existent**
○ Belching   ○ Upper abdominal pain and discomfort
○ Nausea   ○ Difficulty or pain with swallowing
○ Stomach fullness or bloating   ○ Wheezing or dry cough

Other symptoms: _____

Post-lunch energy level: ○ low ○ medium ○ high

Dinner

Time: _____

List the foods you ate for dinner.

_____   _____

_____   _____

_____   _____

Drink _____   **Drink** _____
○ room-temp ○ hot ○ cold   ○ room-temp ○ hot ○ cold

Comments: _____

Physical symptoms after meal: ○ **low** ○ **intense** ○ **non-existent**
○ Belching   ○ Upper abdominal pain and discomfort
○ Nausea   ○ Difficulty or pain with swallowing
○ Stomach fullness or bloating ○ Wheezing or dry cough

Other symptoms: _____

Post-dinner energy level: ○ low ○ medium ○ high

Snack

Time: _____

List the foods you ate as a snack.

_____   _____

Drink _____ ○ room-temp ○ hot ○ cold

Comments: _____

Post-snack energy level: ○ low ○ medium ○ high

Snack

Time: _____

List the foods you ate as a snack.

_____   _____

Drink _____ ○ room-temp ○ hot ○ cold

Comments: _____

Post-snack energy level: ○ low ○ medium ○ high

Medications & Supplements

Include prescription medication, over-the-counter medication & vitamin supplements.

_____   _____

_____   _____

_____   _____

_____   _____

_____   _____

Energy level | Restfulness

Today's waking energy level?
○ low   ○ medium   ○ high

# of times roused from sleep last night?
○ 1   ○ 2   ○ 3+

Last night's reflux/GERD symptoms:

_____   _____

_____   _____

Bed raised?   ○ Y   ○ N   Wedged Pillows?   ○ Y   ○ N

Last meal time? _____   Approx bedtime? _____ am pm
(Remember to give yourself at least 2-3 hours after meals before lying down.)

End-of-day notes

Noticeable change in symptoms? *(Ex: "Throat discomfort has completely disappeared.")*

_____

_____

New terms to research   Books & websites with helpful info

_____   _____

_____   _____

Additional notes:

_____

_____

_____

Breakfast

Time: _____

List the foods you ate for breakfast.

_____   _____

_____   _____

_____   _____

Drink _____   **Drink** _____
○ room-temp ○ hot ○ cold   ○ room-temp ○ hot ○ cold

Comments:

Physical symptoms after meal: ○ **low** ○ **intense** ○ **non-existent**
○ Belching   ○ Upper abdominal pain and discomfort
○ Nausea   ○ Difficulty or pain with swallowing
○ Stomach fullness or bloating   ○ Wheezing or dry cough

Other symptoms:

Post-breakfast energy level: ○ low ○ medium ○ high

Lunch

Time: _____

List the foods you ate for lunch.

_____   _____

_____   _____

_____   _____

Drink _____   **Drink** _____
○ room-temp ○ hot ○ cold   ○ room-temp ○ hot ○ cold

Comments:

Physical symptoms after meal: ○ **low** ○ **intense** ○ **non-existent**
○ Belching   ○ Upper abdominal pain and discomfort
○ Nausea   ○ Difficulty or pain with swallowing
○ Stomach fullness or bloating   ○ Wheezing or dry cough

Other symptoms:

Post-lunch energy level: ○ low ○ medium ○ high

Dinner

Time: _____

List the foods you ate for dinner.

_____   _____

_____   _____

_____   _____

Drink _____   **Drink** _____
○ room-temp   ○ hot   ○ cold   ○ room-temp   ○ hot   ○ cold

Comments: _____

Physical symptoms after meal: ○ **low**   ○ **intense**   ○ **non-existent**
○ Belching   ○ Upper abdominal pain and discomfort
○ Nausea   ○ Difficulty or pain with swallowing
○ Stomach fullness or bloating   ○ Wheezing or dry cough

Other symptoms: _____

Post-dinner energy level: ○ low   ○ medium   ○ high

Snack

Time: _____

List the foods you ate as a snack.

_____   _____

Drink _____   ○ room-temp   ○ hot   ○ cold

Comments: _____

Post-snack energy level: ○ low   ○ medium   ○ high

Snack

Time: _____

List the foods you ate as a snack.

_____   _____

Drink _____   ○ room-temp   ○ hot   ○ cold

Comments: _____

Post-snack energy level: ○ low   ○ medium   ○ high

Medications & Supplements

Include prescription medication, over-the-counter medication & vitamin supplements.

_____   _____

_____   _____

_____   _____

_____   _____

_____   _____

Energy level | Restfulness

Today's waking energy level?
○ low   ○ medium   ○ high

# of times roused from sleep last night?
○ 1   ○ 2   ○ 3+

Last night's reflux/GERD symptoms:

_____   _____

_____   _____

Bed raised?   ○ Y   ○ N   Wedged Pillows?   ○ Y   ○ N

Last meal time? _____   Approx bedtime? _____   am   pm
(Remember to give yourself at least 2-3 hours after meals before lying down.)

End-of-day notes

Noticeable change in symptoms? *(Ex: "Throat discomfort has completely disappeared.")*

_____

_____

New terms to research   Books & websites with helpful info

_____   _____

Additional notes:

_____

_____

_____

Breakfast   Time: _____

List the foods you ate for breakfast.

_____   _____

_____   _____

_____   _____

Drink _____   **Drink** _____
○ room-temp ○ hot ○ cold   ○ room-temp ○ hot ○ cold

Comments:

Physical symptoms after meal: ○ **low**   ○ **intense**   ○ **non-existent**
○ Belching   ○ Upper abdominal pain and discomfort
○ Nausea   ○ Difficulty or pain with swallowing
○ Stomach fullness or bloating   ○ Wheezing or dry cough

Other symptoms:

Post-breakfast energy level: ○ low   ○ medium   ○ high

Lunch   Time: _____

List the foods you ate for lunch.

_____   _____

_____   _____

_____   _____

Drink _____   **Drink** _____
○ room-temp ○ hot ○ cold   ○ room-temp ○ hot ○ cold

Comments:

Physical symptoms after meal: ○ **low**   ○ **intense**   ○ **non-existent**
○ Belching   ○ Upper abdominal pain and discomfort
○ Nausea   ○ Difficulty or pain with swallowing
○ Stomach fullness or bloating   ○ Wheezing or dry cough

Other symptoms:

Post-lunch energy level: ○ low   ○ medium   ○ high

Dinner

Time: _____

List the foods you ate for dinner.

_____   _____

_____   _____

_____   _____

Drink _____   **Drink** _____
○ room-temp ○ hot ○ cold   ○ room-temp ○ hot ○ cold

Comments: _____

Physical symptoms after meal: ○ **low** ○ **intense** ○ **non-existent**

○ Belching   ○ Upper abdominal pain and discomfort
○ Nausea   ○ Difficulty or pain with swallowing
○ Stomach fullness or bloating ○ Wheezing or dry cough

Other symptoms: _____

Post-dinner energy level: ○ low ○ medium ○ high

Snack

Time: _____

List the foods you ate as a snack.

_____   _____

Drink _____   ○ room-temp ○ hot ○ cold

Comments: _____

Post-snack energy level: ○ low ○ medium ○ high

Snack

Time: _____

List the foods you ate as a snack.

_____   _____

Drink _____   ○ room-temp ○ hot ○ cold

Comments: _____

Post-snack energy level: ○ low ○ medium ○ high

Medications & Supplements

Include prescription medication, over-the-counter medication & vitamin supplements.

_____   _____

_____   _____

_____   _____

_____   _____

_____   _____

Energy level | Restfulness

Today's waking energy level?
○ low   ○ medium   ○ high

# of times roused from sleep last night?
○ 1   ○ 2   ○ 3+

Last night's reflux/GERD symptoms:

_____   _____

_____   _____

Bed raised?   ○ Y   ○ N   Wedged Pillows?   ○ Y   ○ N

Last meal time? _____   Approx bedtime? _____ am pm
(Remember to give yourself at least 2-3 hours after meals before lying down.)

End-of-day notes

Noticeable change in symptoms? _(Ex: "Throat discomfort has completely disappeared.")_

_____

_____

New terms to research   Books & websites with helpful info

_____   _____

_____   _____

Additional notes:

_____

_____

_____

Breakfast

Time: _____

List the foods you ate for breakfast.

_____   _____

_____   _____

_____   _____

Drink _____   **Drink** _____
○ room-temp ○ hot ○ cold   ○ room-temp ○ hot ○ cold

Comments:

Physical symptoms after meal: ○ **low** ○ **intense** ○ **non-existent**
○ Belching   ○ Upper abdominal pain and discomfort
○ Nausea   ○ Difficulty or pain with swallowing
○ Stomach fullness or bloating ○ Wheezing or dry cough

Other symptoms:

Post-breakfast energy level: ○ low ○ medium ○ high

Lunch

Time: _____

List the foods you ate for lunch.

_____   _____

_____   _____

_____   _____

Drink _____   **Drink** _____
○ room-temp ○ hot ○ cold   ○ room-temp ○ hot ○ cold

Comments:

Physical symptoms after meal: ○ **low** ○ **intense** ○ **non-existent**
○ Belching   ○ Upper abdominal pain and discomfort
○ Nausea   ○ Difficulty or pain with swallowing
○ Stomach fullness or bloating ○ Wheezing or dry cough

Other symptoms:

Post-lunch energy level: ○ low ○ medium ○ high

Dinner

Time: _____

List the foods you ate for dinner.

_____   _____

_____   _____

_____   _____

Drink _____   **Drink** _____
○ room-temp ○ hot ○ cold   ○ room-temp ○ hot ○ cold

Comments: _____

Physical symptoms after meal: ○ **low**   ○ **intense**   ○ **non-existent**

○ Belching   ○ Upper abdominal pain and discomfort
○ Nausea   ○ Difficulty or pain with swallowing
○ Stomach fullness or bloating   ○ Wheezing or dry cough

Other symptoms: _____

Post-dinner energy level: ○ low   ○ medium   ○ high

Snack

Time: _____

List the foods you ate as a snack.

_____   _____

Drink _____   ○ room-temp   ○ hot   ○ cold

Comments: _____

Post-snack energy level: ○ low   ○ medium   ○ high

Snack

Time: _____

List the foods you ate as a snack.

_____   _____

Drink _____   ○ room-temp   ○ hot   ○ cold

Comments: _____

Post-snack energy level: ○ low   ○ medium   ○ high

Medications & Supplements

Include prescription medication, over-the-counter medication & vitamin supplements.

_____   _____

_____   _____

_____   _____

_____   _____

_____   _____

Energy level | Restfulness

Today's waking energy level?
○ low   ○ medium   ○ high

# of times roused from sleep last night?
○ 1   ○ 2   ○ 3+

Last night's reflux/GERD symptoms:

_____   _____

_____   _____

Bed raised?   ○ Y   ○ N   Wedged Pillows?   ○ Y   ○ N

Last meal time? _____   Approx bedtime? _____ am pm

(Remember to give yourself at least 2-3 hours after meals before lying down.)

End-of-day notes

Noticeable change in symptoms? *(Ex: "Throat discomfort has completely disappeared.")*

_____

_____

New terms to research   Books & websites with helpful info

_____   _____

_____   _____

Additional notes:

_____

_____

_____

Breakfast   Time: _____

List the foods you ate for breakfast.

_____   _____

_____   _____

_____   _____

Drink _____   **Drink** _____
  ○ room-temp   ○ hot   ○ cold   ○ room-temp   ○ hot   ○ cold

Comments: _____

Physical symptoms after meal: ○ **low**   ○ **intense**   ○ **non-existent**
○ Belching   ○ Upper abdominal pain and discomfort
○ Nausea   ○ Difficulty or pain with swallowing
○ Stomach fullness or bloating   ○ Wheezing or dry cough

Other symptoms: _____

Post-breakfast energy level: ○ low   ○ medium   ○ high

Lunch   Time: _____

List the foods you ate for lunch.

_____   _____

_____   _____

_____   _____

Drink _____   **Drink** _____
  ○ room-temp   ○ hot   ○ cold   ○ room-temp   ○ hot   ○ cold

Comments: _____

Physical symptoms after meal: ○ **low**   ○ **intense**   ○ **non-existent**
○ Belching   ○ Upper abdominal pain and discomfort
○ Nausea   ○ Difficulty or pain with swallowing
○ Stomach fullness or bloating   ○ Wheezing or dry cough

Other symptoms: _____

Post-lunch energy level: ○ low   ○ medium   ○ high

Dinner

Time: _____

List the foods you ate for dinner.

_____   _____

_____   _____

_____   _____

Drink _____   **Drink** _____
○ room-temp ○ hot ○ cold   ○ room-temp ○ hot ○ cold

Comments: _____

Physical symptoms after meal: ○ **low** ○ **intense** ○ **non-existent**

○ Belching   ○ Upper abdominal pain and discomfort
○ Nausea   ○ Difficulty or pain with swallowing
○ Stomach fullness or bloating   ○ Wheezing or dry cough

Other symptoms: _____

Post-dinner energy level: ○ low   ○ medium   ○ high

Snack

Time: _____

List the foods you ate as a snack.

_____   _____

Drink _____   ○ room-temp   ○ hot   ○ cold

Comments: _____

Post-snack energy level: ○ low   ○ medium   ○ high

Snack

Time: _____

List the foods you ate as a snack.

_____   _____

Drink _____   ○ room-temp   ○ hot   ○ cold

Comments: _____

Post-snack energy level: ○ low   ○ medium   ○ high

Medications & Supplements

Include prescription medication, over-the-counter medication & vitamin supplements.

_____   _____

_____   _____

_____   _____

_____   _____

_____   _____

Energy level | Restfulness

Today's waking energy level?
○ low   ○ medium   ○ high

# of times roused from sleep last night?
○ 1   ○ 2   ○ 3+

Last night's reflux/GERD symptoms:

_____   _____

_____   _____

Bed raised?   ○ Y   ○ N   Wedged Pillows?   ○ Y   ○ N

Last meal time? _____   Approx bedtime? _____ am pm
(Remember to give yourself at least 2-3 hours after meals before lying down.)

End-of-day notes

Noticeable change in symptoms? _(Ex: "Throat discomfort has completely disappeared.")_

_____

_____

New terms to research   Books & websites with helpful info

_____   _____

_____   _____

Additional notes:

_____

_____

_____

Breakfast   Time: _____

List the foods you ate for breakfast.

_____   _____

_____   _____

_____   _____

Drink _____   **Drink** _____
○ room-temp ○ hot ○ cold   ○ room-temp ○ hot ○ cold

Comments:

Physical symptoms after meal: ○ **low**   ○ **intense**   ○ **non-existent**
○ Belching   ○ Upper abdominal pain and discomfort
○ Nausea   ○ Difficulty or pain with swallowing
○ Stomach fullness or bloating   ○ Wheezing or dry cough

Other symptoms:

Post-breakfast energy level: ○ low   ○ medium   ○ high

Lunch   Time: _____

List the foods you ate for lunch.

_____   _____

_____   _____

_____   _____

Drink _____   **Drink** _____
○ room-temp ○ hot ○ cold   ○ room-temp ○ hot ○ cold

Comments:

Physical symptoms after meal: ○ **low**   ○ **intense**   ○ **non-existent**
○ Belching   ○ Upper abdominal pain and discomfort
○ Nausea   ○ Difficulty or pain with swallowing
○ Stomach fullness or bloating   ○ Wheezing or dry cough

Other symptoms:

Post-lunch energy level: ○ low   ○ medium   ○ high

Dinner

Time: _____

List the foods you ate for dinner.

_____   _____

_____   _____

_____   _____

Drink _____   **Drink** _____
○ room-temp ○ hot ○ cold   ○ room-temp ○ hot ○ cold

Comments: _____

Physical symptoms after meal: ○ **low** ○ **intense** ○ **non-existent**
○ Belching   ○ Upper abdominal pain and discomfort
○ Nausea   ○ Difficulty or pain with swallowing
○ Stomach fullness or bloating ○ Wheezing or dry cough

Other symptoms: _____

Post-dinner energy level: ○ low ○ medium ○ high

Snack

Time: _____

List the foods you ate as a snack.

_____   _____

Drink _____   ○ room-temp ○ hot ○ cold

Comments: _____

Post-snack energy level: ○ low ○ medium ○ high

Snack

Time: _____

List the foods you ate as a snack.

_____   _____

Drink _____   ○ room-temp ○ hot ○ cold

Comments: _____

Post-snack energy level: ○ low ○ medium ○ high

Medications & Supplements

Include prescription medication, over-the-counter medication & vitamin supplements.

_____   _____

_____   _____

_____   _____

_____   _____

_____   _____

Energy level | Restfulness

Today's waking energy level?
○ low   ○ medium   ○ high

# of times roused from sleep last night?
○ 1   ○ 2   ○ 3+

Last night's reflux/GERD symptoms:

_____   _____

_____   _____

Bed raised?   ○ Y   ○ N   Wedged Pillows?   ○ Y   ○ N

Last meal time? _____   Approx bedtime? _____   am   pm
(Remember to give yourself at least 2-3 hours after meals before lying down.)

End-of-day notes

Noticeable change in symptoms? _(Ex: "Throat discomfort has completely disappeared.")_

_____

_____

New terms to research   Books & websites with helpful info

_____   _____

_____   _____

Additional notes:

_____

_____

_____

_____

Breakfast   Time: _____

List the foods you ate for breakfast.

_____   _____

_____   _____

_____   _____

Drink _____   **Drink** _____
○ room-temp ○ hot ○ cold   ○ room-temp ○ hot ○ cold

Comments:
_____

Physical symptoms after meal: ○ **low**   ○ **intense**   ○ **non-existent**
○ Belching   ○ Upper abdominal pain and discomfort
○ Nausea   ○ Difficulty or pain with swallowing
○ Stomach fullness or bloating   ○ Wheezing or dry cough

Other symptoms:
_____

Post-breakfast energy level: ○ low   ○ medium   ○ high

Lunch   Time: _____

List the foods you ate for lunch.

_____   _____

_____   _____

_____   _____

Drink _____   **Drink** _____
○ room-temp ○ hot ○ cold   ○ room-temp ○ hot ○ cold

Comments:
_____

Physical symptoms after meal: ○ **low**   ○ **intense**   ○ **non-existent**
○ Belching   ○ Upper abdominal pain and discomfort
○ Nausea   ○ Difficulty or pain with swallowing
○ Stomach fullness or bloating   ○ Wheezing or dry cough

Other symptoms:
_____

Post-lunch energy level: ○ low   ○ medium   ○ high

Dinner

Time: _____

List the foods you ate for dinner.

_____   _____

_____   _____

_____   _____

Drink _____ ○ room-temp ○ hot ○ cold

Drink _____ ○ room-temp ○ hot ○ cold

Comments: _____

Physical symptoms after meal: ○ **low** ○ **intense** ○ **non-existent**

○ Belching   ○ Upper abdominal pain and discomfort
○ Nausea   ○ Difficulty or pain with swallowing
○ Stomach fullness or bloating ○ Wheezing or dry cough

Other symptoms: _____

Post-dinner energy level: ○ low ○ medium ○ high

Snack

Time: _____

List the foods you ate as a snack.

_____   _____

Drink _____   ○ room-temp ○ hot ○ cold

Comments: _____

Post-snack energy level: ○ low ○ medium ○ high

Snack

Time: _____

List the foods you ate as a snack.

_____   _____

Drink _____   ○ room-temp ○ hot ○ cold

Comments: _____

Post-snack energy level: ○ low ○ medium ○ high

Medications & Supplements

Include prescription medication, over-the-counter medication & vitamin supplements.

_____   _____

_____   _____

_____   _____

_____   _____

_____   _____

Energy level | Restfulness

Today's waking energy level?
○ low   ○ medium   ○ high

# of times roused from sleep last night?
○ 1   ○ 2   ○ 3+

Last night's reflux/GERD symptoms:

_____   _____

_____   _____

Bed raised?   ○ Y   ○ N   Wedged Pillows?   ○ Y   ○ N

Last meal time? _____   Approx bedtime? _____ am pm
(Remember to give yourself at least 2-3 hours after meals before lying down.)

End-of-day notes

Noticeable change in symptoms? _(Ex: "Throat discomfort has completely disappeared.")_

_____

_____

New terms to research   Books & websites with helpful info

_____   _____

_____   _____

Additional notes:

_____

_____

_____

Breakfast

Time: _____

List the foods you ate for breakfast.

_____   _____

_____   _____

_____   _____

Drink _____   **Drink** _____
   ○ room-temp ○ hot ○ cold   ○ room-temp ○ hot ○ cold

Comments:

Physical symptoms after meal: ○ **low** ○ **intense** ○ **non-existent**
○ Belching   ○ Upper abdominal pain and discomfort
○ Nausea   ○ Difficulty or pain with swallowing
○ Stomach fullness or bloating ○ Wheezing or dry cough

Other symptoms:

Post-breakfast energy level: ○ low ○ medium ○ high

Lunch

Time: _____

List the foods you ate for lunch.

_____   _____

_____   _____

_____   _____

Drink _____   **Drink** _____
   ○ room-temp ○ hot ○ cold   ○ room-temp ○ hot ○ cold

Comments:

Physical symptoms after meal: ○ **low** ○ **intense** ○ **non-existent**
○ Belching   ○ Upper abdominal pain and discomfort
○ Nausea   ○ Difficulty or pain with swallowing
○ Stomach fullness or bloating ○ Wheezing or dry cough

Other symptoms:

Post-lunch energy level: ○ low ○ medium ○ high

Dinner

Time: _____

List the foods you ate for dinner.

_____   _____

_____   _____

_____   _____

Drink _____   **Drink** _____
○ room-temp ○ hot ○ cold   ○ room-temp ○ hot ○ cold

Comments: _____

Physical symptoms after meal: ○ **low** ○ **intense** ○ **non-existent**
○ Belching   ○ Upper abdominal pain and discomfort
○ Nausea   ○ Difficulty or pain with swallowing
○ Stomach fullness or bloating ○ Wheezing or dry cough

Other symptoms: _____

Post-dinner energy level: ○ low ○ medium ○ high

Snack

Time: _____

List the foods you ate as a snack.

_____   _____

Drink _____ ○ room-temp ○ hot ○ cold

Comments: _____

Post-snack energy level: ○ low ○ medium ○ high

Snack

Time: _____

List the foods you ate as a snack.

_____   _____

Drink _____ ○ room-temp ○ hot ○ cold

Comments: _____

Post-snack energy level: ○ low ○ medium ○ high

Medications & Supplements

Include prescription medication, over-the-counter medication & vitamin supplements.

_____   _____

_____   _____

_____   _____

_____   _____

_____   _____

Energy level | Restfulness

Today's waking energy level?
○ low   ○ medium   ○ high

# of times roused from sleep last night?
○ 1   ○ 2   ○ 3+

Last night's reflux/GERD symptoms:

_____   _____

_____   _____

Bed raised?   ○ Y   ○ N   Wedged Pillows?   ○ Y   ○ N

Last meal time? _____   Approx bedtime? _____ am pm
(Remember to give yourself at least 2-3 hours after meals before lying down.)

End-of-day notes

Noticeable change in symptoms? *(Ex: "Throat discomfort has completely disappeared.")*

_____

_____

New terms to research   Books & websites with helpful info

_____   _____

_____   _____

Additional notes:

_____

_____

_____

Breakfast   Time: _____

List the foods you ate for breakfast.

_____   _____

_____   _____

                                 _____

Drink _____   **Drink** _____
○ room-temp ○ hot ○ cold   ○ room-temp ○ hot ○ cold

Comments:
_____

Physical symptoms after meal: ○ **low**   ○ **intense**   ○ **non-existent**
○ Belching   ○ Upper abdominal pain and discomfort
○ Nausea   ○ Difficulty or pain with swallowing
○ Stomach fullness or bloating   ○ Wheezing or dry cough

Other symptoms:
_____

Post-breakfast energy level: ○ low   ○ medium   ○ high

Lunch   Time: _____

List the foods you ate for lunch.

_____   _____

_____   _____

                                 _____

Drink _____   **Drink** _____
○ room-temp ○ hot ○ cold   ○ room-temp ○ hot ○ cold

Comments:
_____

Physical symptoms after meal: ○ **low**   ○ **intense**   ○ **non-existent**
○ Belching   ○ Upper abdominal pain and discomfort
○ Nausea   ○ Difficulty or pain with swallowing
○ Stomach fullness or bloating   ○ Wheezing or dry cough

Other symptoms:
_____

Post-lunch energy level: ○ low   ○ medium   ○ high

Dinner

Time: _____

List the foods you ate for dinner.

_____   _____

_____   _____

_____   _____

Drink _____   **Drink** _____
○ room-temp   ○ hot   ○ cold   ○ room-temp   ○ hot   ○ cold

Comments: _____

Physical symptoms after meal: ○ **low**   ○ **intense**   ○ **non-existent**
○ Belching   ○ Upper abdominal pain and discomfort
○ Nausea   ○ Difficulty or pain with swallowing
○ Stomach fullness or bloating   ○ Wheezing or dry cough

Other symptoms: _____

Post-dinner energy level: ○ low   ○ medium   ○ high

Snack

Time: _____

List the foods you ate as a snack.

_____   _____

Drink _____   ○ room-temp   ○ hot   ○ cold

Comments: _____

Post-snack energy level: ○ low   ○ medium   ○ high

Snack

Time: _____

List the foods you ate as a snack.

_____   _____

Drink _____   ○ room-temp   ○ hot   ○ cold

Comments: _____

Post-snack energy level: ○ low   ○ medium   ○ high

Medications & Supplements

Include prescription medication, over-the-counter medication & vitamin supplements.

_____   _____

_____   _____

_____   _____

_____   _____

_____   _____

Energy level | Restfulness

Today's waking energy level?
○ low   ○ medium   ○ high

# of times roused from sleep last night?
○ 1   ○ 2   ○ 3+

Last night's reflux/GERD symptoms:

_____   _____

_____   _____

Bed raised?   ○ Y   ○ N   Wedged Pillows?   ○ Y   ○ N

Last meal time? _____   Approx bedtime? _____   am   pm
(Remember to give yourself at least 2-3 hours after meals before lying down.)

End-of-day notes

Noticeable change in symptoms? *(Ex: "Throat discomfort has completely disappeared.")*

_____

_____

New terms to research   Books & websites with helpful info

_____   _____

_____   _____

Additional notes:

_____

_____

_____

Breakfast
Time: _____

List the foods you ate for breakfast.

_____   _____

_____   _____

_____   _____

Drink _____   **Drink** _____
○ room-temp   ○ hot   ○ cold   ○ room-temp   ○ hot   ○ cold

Comments:
_____

Physical symptoms after meal: ○ **low**   ○ **intense**   ○ **non-existent**

○ Belching   ○ Upper abdominal pain and discomfort
○ Nausea   ○ Difficulty or pain with swallowing
○ Stomach fullness or bloating ○ Wheezing or dry cough

Other symptoms:
_____

Post-breakfast energy level: ○ low   ○ medium   ○ high

Lunch
Time: _____

List the foods you ate for lunch.

_____   _____

_____   _____

_____   _____

Drink _____   **Drink** _____
○ room-temp   ○ hot   ○ cold   ○ room-temp   ○ hot   ○ cold

Comments:
_____

Physical symptoms after meal: ○ **low**   ○ **intense**   ○ **non-existent**

○ Belching   ○ Upper abdominal pain and discomfort
○ Nausea   ○ Difficulty or pain with swallowing
○ Stomach fullness or bloating ○ Wheezing or dry cough

Other symptoms:
_____

Post-lunch energy level: ○ low   ○ medium   ○ high

Dinner

Time: _____

List the foods you ate for dinner.

_____   _____

_____   _____

_____   _____

Drink _____   **Drink** _____
○ room-temp ○ hot ○ cold   ○ room-temp ○ hot ○ cold

Comments: _____

Physical symptoms after meal: ○ **low** ○ **intense** ○ **non-existent**
○ Belching   ○ Upper abdominal pain and discomfort
○ Nausea   ○ Difficulty or pain with swallowing
○ Stomach fullness or bloating   ○ Wheezing or dry cough

Other symptoms: _____

Post-dinner energy level: ○ low ○ medium ○ high

Snack

Time: _____

List the foods you ate as a snack.

_____   _____

Drink _____   ○ room-temp ○ hot ○ cold

Comments: _____

Post-snack energy level: ○ low ○ medium ○ high

Snack

Time: _____

List the foods you ate as a snack.

_____   _____

Drink _____   ○ room-temp ○ hot ○ cold

Comments: _____

Post-snack energy level: ○ low ○ medium ○ high

Medications & Supplements

Include prescription medication, over-the-counter medication & vitamin supplements.

_____   _____

_____   _____

_____   _____

_____   _____

_____   _____

Energy level | Restfulness

Today's waking energy level?
○ low   ○ medium   ○ high

# of times roused from sleep last night?
○ 1   ○ 2   ○ 3+

Last night's reflux/GERD symptoms:

_____   _____

_____   _____

Bed raised?   ○ Y   ○ N   Wedged Pillows?   ○ Y   ○ N

Last meal time? _____   Approx bedtime? _____   am   pm
(Remember to give yourself at least 2-3 hours after meals before lying down.)

End-of-day notes

Noticeable change in symptoms? _(Ex: "Throat discomfort has completely disappeared.")_

_____

_____

New terms to research   Books & websites with helpful info

_____   _____

_____   _____

Additional notes:

_____

_____

_____

_____

Breakfast

Time: _____

List the foods you ate for breakfast.

_____   _____

_____   _____

_____   _____

Drink _____   **Drink** _____
○ room-temp   ○ hot   ○ cold   ○ room-temp   ○ hot   ○ cold

Comments: _____

Physical symptoms after meal: ○ **low**   ○ **intense**   ○ **non-existent**
○ Belching   ○ Upper abdominal pain and discomfort
○ Nausea   ○ Difficulty or pain with swallowing
○ Stomach fullness or bloating   ○ Wheezing or dry cough

Other symptoms: _____

Post-breakfast energy level: ○ low   ○ medium   ○ high

Lunch

Time: _____

List the foods you ate for lunch.

_____   _____

_____   _____

_____   _____

Drink _____   **Drink** _____
○ room-temp   ○ hot   ○ cold   ○ room-temp   ○ hot   ○ cold

Comments: _____

Physical symptoms after meal: ○ **low**   ○ **intense**   ○ **non-existent**
○ Belching   ○ Upper abdominal pain and discomfort
○ Nausea   ○ Difficulty or pain with swallowing
○ Stomach fullness or bloating   ○ Wheezing or dry cough

Other symptoms: _____

Post-lunch energy level: ○ low   ○ medium   ○ high

Dinner

Time: _____

List the foods you ate for dinner.

_____ _____

_____ _____

_____ _____

Drink _____ **Drink** _____
   ○ room-temp ○ hot ○ cold   ○ room-temp ○ hot ○ cold

Comments: _____

Physical symptoms after meal: ○ **low** ○ **intense** ○ **non-existent**
○ Belching ○ Upper abdominal pain and discomfort
○ Nausea ○ Difficulty or pain with swallowing
○ Stomach fullness or bloating ○ Wheezing or dry cough

Other symptoms: _____

Post-dinner energy level: ○ low ○ medium ○ high

Snack

Time: _____

List the foods you ate as a snack.

_____ _____

Drink _____ ○ room-temp ○ hot ○ cold

Comments: _____

Post-snack energy level: ○ low ○ medium ○ high

Snack

Time: _____

List the foods you ate as a snack.

_____ _____

Drink _____ ○ room-temp ○ hot ○ cold

Comments: _____

Post-snack energy level: ○ low ○ medium ○ high

Medications & Supplements

Include prescription medication, over-the-counter medication & vitamin supplements.

_____   _____

_____   _____

_____   _____

_____   _____

_____   _____

Energy level | Restfulness

Today's waking energy level?
○ low   ○ medium   ○ high

# of times roused from sleep last night?
○ 1   ○ 2   ○ 3+

Last night's reflux/GERD symptoms:

_____   _____

_____   _____

Bed raised?   ○ Y   ○ N   Wedged Pillows?   ○ Y   ○ N

Last meal time? _____   Approx bedtime? _____ am   pm
(Remember to give yourself at least 2-3 hours after meals before lying down.)

End-of-day notes

Noticeable change in symptoms? _(Ex: "Throat discomfort has completely disappeared.")_

_____

_____

New terms to research   Books & websites with helpful info

_____   _____

_____   _____

Additional notes:

_____

_____

_____

Breakfast   Time: _____

List the foods you ate for breakfast.

_____   _____

_____   _____

_____   _____

Drink _____   **Drink** _____
○ room-temp ○ hot ○ cold   ○ room-temp ○ hot ○ cold

Physical symptoms after meal: ○ **low** ○ **intense** ○ **non-existent**
○ Belching   ○ Upper abdominal pain and discomfort
○ Nausea   ○ Difficulty or pain with swallowing
○ Stomach fullness or bloating ○ Wheezing or dry cough

Other symptoms:

Post-breakfast energy level: ○ low ○ medium ○ high

Lunch   Time: _____

List the foods you ate for lunch.

_____   _____

_____   _____

_____   _____

Drink _____   **Drink** _____
○ room-temp ○ hot ○ cold   ○ room-temp ○ hot ○ cold

Comments:

Physical symptoms after meal: ○ **low** ○ **intense** ○ **non-existent**
○ Belching   ○ Upper abdominal pain and discomfort
○ Nausea   ○ Difficulty or pain with swallowing
○ Stomach fullness or bloating ○ Wheezing or dry cough

Other symptoms:

Post-lunch energy level: ○ low ○ medium ○ high

Dinner

Time: _____

List the foods you ate for dinner.

_____   _____

_____   _____

_____   _____

Drink _____   **Drink** _____
  ○ room-temp ○ hot ○ cold   ○ room-temp ○ hot ○ cold

Comments: _____

Physical symptoms after meal: ○ **low**   ○ **intense**   ○ **non-existent**
○ Belching   ○ Upper abdominal pain and discomfort
○ Nausea   ○ Difficulty or pain with swallowing
○ Stomach fullness or bloating   ○ Wheezing or dry cough

Other symptoms: _____

Post-dinner energy level: ○ low   ○ medium   ○ high

Snack

Time: _____

List the foods you ate as a snack.

_____   _____

Drink _____   ○ room-temp   ○ hot   ○ cold

Comments: _____

Post-snack energy level: ○ low   ○ medium   ○ high

Snack

Time: _____

List the foods you ate as a snack.

_____   _____

Drink _____   ○ room-temp   ○ hot   ○ cold

Comments: _____

Post-snack energy level: ○ low   ○ medium   ○ high

Medications & Supplements

Include prescription medication, over-the-counter medication & vitamin supplements.

_____   _____

_____   _____

_____   _____

_____   _____

_____   _____

Energy level | Restfulness

Today's waking energy level?
○ low   ○ medium   ○ high

# of times roused from sleep last night?
○ 1   ○ 2   ○ 3+

Last night's reflux/GERD symptoms:

_____   _____

_____   _____

Bed raised?   ○ Y   ○ N   Wedged Pillows?   ○ Y   ○ N

Last meal time? _____   Approx bedtime? _____ am pm
(Remember to give yourself at least 2-3 hours after meals before lying down.)

End-of-day notes

Noticeable change in symptoms? _(Ex: "Throat discomfort has completely disappeared.")_

_____

_____

New terms to research   Books & websites with helpful info

_____   _____

_____   _____

Additional notes:

_____

_____

_____

Breakfast   Time: _____

List the foods you ate for breakfast.

_____   _____

_____   _____

_____   _____

Drink _____   **Drink** _____
○ room-temp ○ hot ○ cold   ○ room-temp ○ hot ○ cold

Comments: _____

Physical symptoms after meal: ○ **low**   ○ **intense**   ○ **non-existent**
○ Belching   ○ Upper abdominal pain and discomfort
○ Nausea   ○ Difficulty or pain with swallowing
○ Stomach fullness or bloating   ○ Wheezing or dry cough

Other symptoms: _____

Post-breakfast energy level: ○ low   ○ medium   ○ high

Lunch   Time: _____

List the foods you ate for lunch.

_____   _____

_____   _____

_____   _____

Drink _____   **Drink** _____
○ room-temp ○ hot ○ cold   ○ room-temp ○ hot ○ cold

Comments: _____

Physical symptoms after meal: ○ **low**   ○ **intense**   ○ **non-existent**
○ Belching   ○ Upper abdominal pain and discomfort
○ Nausea   ○ Difficulty or pain with swallowing
○ Stomach fullness or bloating   ○ Wheezing or dry cough

Other symptoms: _____

Post-lunch energy level: ○ low   ○ medium   ○ high

Dinner

Time: _____

List the foods you ate for dinner.

_____   _____

_____   _____

_____   _____

Drink _____   **Drink** _____
    ○ room-temp ○ hot ○ cold   ○ room-temp ○ hot ○ cold

Comments: _____

Physical symptoms after meal: ○ **low** ○ **intense** ○ **non-existent**
○ Belching   ○ Upper abdominal pain and discomfort
○ Nausea   ○ Difficulty or pain with swallowing
○ Stomach fullness or bloating ○ Wheezing or dry cough

Other symptoms: _____

Post-dinner energy level: ○ low ○ medium ○ high

Snack

Time: _____

List the foods you ate as a snack.

_____   _____

Drink _____ ○ room-temp ○ hot ○ cold

Comments: _____

Post-snack energy level: ○ low ○ medium ○ high

Snack

Time: _____

List the foods you ate as a snack.

_____   _____

Drink _____ ○ room-temp ○ hot ○ cold

Comments: _____

Post-snack energy level: ○ low ○ medium ○ high

Medications & Supplements

Include prescription medication, over-the-counter medication & vitamin supplements.

_____   _____

_____   _____

_____   _____

_____   _____

_____   _____

Energy level | Restfulness

Today's waking energy level?
○ low   ○ medium   ○ high

# of times roused from sleep last night?
○ 1   ○ 2   ○ 3+

Last night's reflux/GERD symptoms:

_____   _____

_____   _____

Bed raised?   ○ Y   ○ N   Wedged Pillows?   ○ Y   ○ N

Last meal time? _____   Approx bedtime? _____   am   pm
(Remember to give yourself at least 2-3 hours after meals before lying down.)

End-of-day notes

Noticeable change in symptoms? *(Ex: "Throat discomfort has completely disappeared.")*

_____

_____

New terms to research   Books & websites with helpful info

_____   _____

_____   _____

Additional notes:

_____

_____

_____

Breakfast
Time: _____

List the foods you ate for breakfast.

_____   _____

_____   _____

_____   _____

Drink _____   **Drink** _____
○ room-temp   ○ hot   ○ cold   ○ room-temp   ○ hot   ○ cold

Comments:

Physical symptoms after meal: ○ **low**   ○ **intense**   ○ **non-existent**
○ Belching   ○ Upper abdominal pain and discomfort
○ Nausea   ○ Difficulty or pain with swallowing
○ Stomach fullness or bloating   ○ Wheezing or dry cough

Other symptoms:

Post-breakfast energy level: ○ low   ○ medium   ○ high

Lunch
Time: _____

List the foods you ate for lunch.

_____   _____

_____   _____

_____   _____

Drink _____   **Drink** _____
○ room-temp   ○ hot   ○ cold   ○ room-temp   ○ hot   ○ cold

Comments:

Physical symptoms after meal: ○ **low**   ○ **intense**   ○ **non-existent**
○ Belching   ○ Upper abdominal pain and discomfort
○ Nausea   ○ Difficulty or pain with swallowing
○ Stomach fullness or bloating   ○ Wheezing or dry cough

Other symptoms:

Post-lunch energy level: ○ low   ○ medium   ○ high

Dinner

Time: _____

List the foods you ate for dinner.

_____   _____

_____   _____

_____   _____

Drink _____   **Drink** _____
○ room-temp ○ hot ○ cold   ○ room-temp ○ hot ○ cold

Comments: _____

Physical symptoms after meal: ○ **low**   ○ **intense**   ○ **non-existent**
○ Belching   ○ Upper abdominal pain and discomfort
○ Nausea   ○ Difficulty or pain with swallowing
○ Stomach fullness or bloating   ○ Wheezing or dry cough

Other symptoms: _____

Post-dinner energy level: ○ low   ○ medium   ○ high

Snack

Time: _____

List the foods you ate as a snack.

_____   _____

Drink _____   ○ room-temp   ○ hot   ○ cold

Comments: _____

Post-snack energy level: ○ low   ○ medium   ○ high

Snack

Time: _____

List the foods you ate as a snack.

_____   _____

Drink _____   ○ room-temp   ○ hot   ○ cold

Comments: _____

Post-snack energy level: ○ low   ○ medium   ○ high

Medications & Supplements

Include prescription medication, over-the-counter medication & vitamin supplements.

_____   _____

_____   _____

_____   _____

_____   _____

_____   _____

Energy level | Restfulness

Today's waking energy level?
○ low   ○ medium   ○ high

# of times roused from sleep last night?
○ 1   ○ 2   ○ 3+

Last night's reflux/GERD symptoms:

_____   _____

_____   _____

Bed raised?   ○ Y   ○ N   Wedged Pillows?   ○ Y   ○ N

Last meal time? _____   Approx bedtime? _____ am pm
(Remember to give yourself at least 2-3 hours after meals before lying down.)

End-of-day notes

Noticeable change in symptoms? *(Ex: "Throat discomfort has completely disappeared.")*

_____

_____

New terms to research   Books & websites with helpful info

_____   _____

_____   _____

Additional notes:

_____

_____

_____

Breakfast   Time: _____

List the foods you ate for breakfast.

_____   _____

_____   _____

_____   _____

Drink _____   **Drink** _____
○ room-temp   ○ hot   ○ cold   ○ room-temp   ○ hot   ○ cold

Comments: _____

Physical symptoms after meal: ○ **low**   ○ **intense**   ○ **non-existent**
○ Belching   ○ Upper abdominal pain and discomfort
○ Nausea   ○ Difficulty or pain with swallowing
○ Stomach fullness or bloating   ○ Wheezing or dry cough

Other symptoms: _____

Post-breakfast energy level: ○ low   ○ medium   ○ high

Lunch   Time: _____

List the foods you ate for lunch.

_____   _____

_____   _____

_____   _____

Drink _____   **Drink** _____
○ room-temp   ○ hot   ○ cold   ○ room-temp   ○ hot   ○ cold

Comments: _____

Physical symptoms after meal: ○ **low**   ○ **intense**   ○ **non-existent**
○ Belching   ○ Upper abdominal pain and discomfort
○ Nausea   ○ Difficulty or pain with swallowing
○ Stomach fullness or bloating   ○ Wheezing or dry cough

Other symptoms: _____

Post-lunch energy level: ○ low   ○ medium   ○ high

Dinner

Time: _____

List the foods you ate for dinner.

_____   _____

_____   _____

_____   _____

Drink _____   **Drink** _____
  ○ room-temp ○ hot ○ cold   ○ room-temp ○ hot ○ cold

Comments: _____

Physical symptoms after meal: ○ **low** ○ **intense** ○ **non-existent**
  ○ Belching   ○ Upper abdominal pain and discomfort
  ○ Nausea   ○ Difficulty or pain with swallowing
  ○ Stomach fullness or bloating ○ Wheezing or dry cough

Other symptoms: _____

Post-dinner energy level: ○ low ○ medium ○ high

Snack

Time: _____

List the foods you ate as a snack.

_____   _____

Drink _____   ○ room-temp ○ hot ○ cold

Comments: _____

Post-snack energy level: ○ low ○ medium ○ high

Snack

Time: _____

List the foods you ate as a snack.

_____   _____

Drink _____   ○ room-temp ○ hot ○ cold

Comments: _____

Post-snack energy level: ○ low ○ medium ○ high

Medications & Supplements

Include prescription medication, over-the-counter medication & vitamin supplements.

_____   _____

_____   _____

_____   _____

_____   _____

_____   _____

Energy level | Restfulness

Today's waking energy level?
○ low   ○ medium   ○ high

# of times roused from sleep last night?
○ 1   ○ 2   ○ 3+

Last night's reflux/GERD symptoms:

_____   _____

_____   _____

Bed raised?   ○ Y   ○ N   Wedged Pillows?   ○ Y   ○ N

Last meal time? _____   Approx bedtime? _____   am   pm
(Remember to give yourself at least 2-3 hours after meals before lying down.)

End-of-day notes

Noticeable change in symptoms? *(Ex: "Throat discomfort has completely disappeared.")*

_____

_____

New terms to research   Books & websites with helpful info

_____   _____

_____   _____

Additional notes:

_____

_____

_____

Breakfast   Time: _____

List the foods you ate for breakfast.

_____   _____

_____   _____

_____   _____

Drink _____   **Drink** _____
   ○ room-temp   ○ hot   ○ cold   ○ room-temp   ○ hot   ○ cold

Comments: _____

Physical symptoms after meal: ○ **low**   ○ **intense**   ○ **non-existent**
○ Belching   ○ Upper abdominal pain and discomfort
○ Nausea   ○ Difficulty or pain with swallowing
○ Stomach fullness or bloating   ○ Wheezing or dry cough

Other symptoms: _____

Post-breakfast energy level: ○ low   ○ medium   ○ high

Lunch   Time: _____

List the foods you ate for lunch.

_____   _____

_____   _____

_____   _____

Drink _____   **Drink** _____
   ○ room-temp   ○ hot   ○ cold   ○ room-temp   ○ hot   ○ cold

Comments: _____

Physical symptoms after meal: ○ **low**   ○ **intense**   ○ **non-existent**
○ Belching   ○ Upper abdominal pain and discomfort
○ Nausea   ○ Difficulty or pain with swallowing
○ Stomach fullness or bloating   ○ Wheezing or dry cough

Other symptoms: _____

Post-lunch energy level: ○ low   ○ medium   ○ high

Dinner

Time: _____

List the foods you ate for dinner.

_____   _____

_____   _____

_____   _____

Drink _____   **Drink** _____
  ○ room-temp ○ hot ○ cold   ○ room-temp ○ hot ○ cold

Comments: _____

Physical symptoms after meal: ○ **low** ○ **intense** ○ **non-existent**
○ Belching   ○ Upper abdominal pain and discomfort
○ Nausea   ○ Difficulty or pain with swallowing
○ Stomach fullness or bloating ○ Wheezing or dry cough

Other symptoms: _____

Post-dinner energy level: ○ low ○ medium ○ high

Snack

Time: _____

List the foods you ate as a snack.

_____   _____

Drink _____   ○ room-temp ○ hot ○ cold

Comments: _____

Post-snack energy level: ○ low ○ medium ○ high

Snack

Time: _____

List the foods you ate as a snack.

_____   _____

Drink _____   ○ room-temp ○ hot ○ cold

Comments: _____

Post-snack energy level: ○ low ○ medium ○ high

Medications & Supplements

Include prescription medication, over-the-counter medication & vitamin supplements.

_____   _____

_____   _____

_____   _____

_____   _____

_____   _____

Energy level | Restfulness

Today's waking energy level?
○ low   ○ medium   ○ high

# of times roused from sleep last night?
○ 1   ○ 2   ○ 3+

Last night's reflux/GERD symptoms:

_____   _____

_____   _____

Bed raised?   ○ Y   ○ N   Wedged Pillows?   ○ Y   ○ N

Last meal time? _____   Approx bedtime? _____   am   pm
(Remember to give yourself at least 2-3 hours after meals before lying down.)

End-of-day notes

Noticeable change in symptoms? *(Ex: "Throat discomfort has completely disappeared.")*

_____

_____

New terms to research   Books & websites with helpful info

_____   _____

_____   _____

Additional notes:

_____

_____

_____

Breakfast   Time: _____

List the foods you ate for breakfast.

_____   _____

_____   _____

_____   _____

Drink _____   **Drink** _____
○ room-temp ○ hot ○ cold   ○ room-temp ○ hot ○ cold

Comments: _____

Physical symptoms after meal: ○ **low** ○ **intense** ○ **non-existent**
○ Belching   ○ Upper abdominal pain and discomfort
○ Nausea   ○ Difficulty or pain with swallowing
○ Stomach fullness or bloating   ○ Wheezing or dry cough

Other symptoms: _____

Post-breakfast energy level: ○ low   ○ medium   ○ high

Lunch   Time: _____

List the foods you ate for lunch.

_____   _____

_____   _____

_____   _____

Drink _____   **Drink** _____
○ room-temp ○ hot ○ cold   ○ room-temp ○ hot ○ cold

Comments: _____

Physical symptoms after meal: ○ **low** ○ **intense** ○ **non-existent**
○ Belching   ○ Upper abdominal pain and discomfort
○ Nausea   ○ Difficulty or pain with swallowing
○ Stomach fullness or bloating   ○ Wheezing or dry cough

Other symptoms: _____

Post-lunch energy level: ○ low   ○ medium   ○ high

Dinner

Time: _____

List the foods you ate for dinner.

_____   _____

_____   _____

_____   _____

Drink _____   **Drink** _____
○ room-temp ○ hot ○ cold   ○ room-temp ○ hot ○ cold

Comments: _____

Physical symptoms after meal: ○ **low**   ○ **intense**   ○ **non-existent**
○ Belching   ○ Upper abdominal pain and discomfort
○ Nausea   ○ Difficulty or pain with swallowing
○ Stomach fullness or bloating   ○ Wheezing or dry cough

Other symptoms: _____

Post-dinner energy level: ○ low   ○ medium   ○ high

Snack

Time: _____

List the foods you ate as a snack.

_____   _____

Drink _____   ○ room-temp   ○ hot   ○ cold

Comments: _____

Post-snack energy level: ○ low   ○ medium   ○ high

Snack

Time: _____

List the foods you ate as a snack.

_____   _____

Drink _____   ○ room-temp   ○ hot   ○ cold

Comments: _____

Post-snack energy level: ○ low   ○ medium   ○ high

Medications & Supplements

Include prescription medication, over-the-counter medication & vitamin supplements.

_____   _____

_____   _____

_____   _____

_____   _____

_____   _____

Energy level | Restfulness

Today's waking energy level?
○ low   ○ medium   ○ high

# of times roused from sleep last night?
○ 1   ○ 2   ○ 3+

Last night's reflux/GERD symptoms:

_____   _____

_____   _____

Bed raised?   ○ Y   ○ N   Wedged Pillows?   ○ Y   ○ N

Last meal time? _____   Approx bedtime? _____   am   pm
    (Remember to give yourself at least 2-3 hours after meals before lying down.)

End-of-day notes

Noticeable change in symptoms? *(Ex: "Throat discomfort has completely disappeared.")*

_____

_____

New terms to research   Books & websites with helpful info

_____   _____

Additional notes:

_____

_____

_____

Breakfast
Time: _____

List the foods you ate for breakfast.

_____ _____

_____ _____

_____ _____

Drink _____ **Drink** _____
○ room-temp ○ hot ○ cold ○ room-temp ○ hot ○ cold

Comments:

Physical symptoms after meal: ○ **low** ○ **intense** ○ **non-existent**
○ Belching ○ Upper abdominal pain and discomfort
○ Nausea ○ Difficulty or pain with swallowing
○ Stomach fullness or bloating ○ Wheezing or dry cough

Other symptoms:

Post-breakfast energy level: ○ low ○ medium ○ high

Lunch
Time: _____

List the foods you ate for lunch.

_____ _____

_____ _____

_____ _____

Drink _____ **Drink** _____
○ room-temp ○ hot ○ cold ○ room-temp ○ hot ○ cold

Comments:

Physical symptoms after meal: ○ **low** ○ **intense** ○ **non-existent**
○ Belching ○ Upper abdominal pain and discomfort
○ Nausea ○ Difficulty or pain with swallowing
○ Stomach fullness or bloating ○ Wheezing or dry cough

Other symptoms:

Post-lunch energy level: ○ low ○ medium ○ high

Dinner

Time: _____

List the foods you ate for dinner.

_____ _____

_____ _____

_____ _____

Drink _____ **Drink** _____
   ○ room-temp ○ hot ○ cold   ○ room-temp ○ hot ○ cold

Comments:
_____

Physical symptoms after meal: ○ **low**   ○ **intense**   ○ **non-existent**
○ Belching   ○ Upper abdominal pain and discomfort
○ Nausea   ○ Difficulty or pain with swallowing
○ Stomach fullness or bloating ○ Wheezing or dry cough

Other symptoms:

Post-dinner energy level: ○ low   ○ medium   ○ high

Snack

Time: _____

List the foods you ate as a snack.

_____ _____

Drink _____   ○ room-temp   ○ hot   ○ cold

Comments: _____

Post-snack energy level: ○ low   ○ medium   ○ high

Snack

Time: _____

List the foods you ate as a snack.

_____ _____

Drink _____   ○ room-temp   ○ hot   ○ cold

Comments: _____

Post-snack energy level: ○ low   ○ medium   ○ high

Medications & Supplements

Include prescription medication, over-the-counter medication & vitamin supplements.

_____   _____

_____   _____

_____   _____

_____   _____

_____   _____

Energy level | Restfulness

Today's waking energy level?
○ low   ○ medium   ○ high

# of times roused from sleep last night?
○ 1   ○ 2   ○ 3+

Last night's reflux/GERD symptoms:

_____   _____

_____   _____

Bed raised?   ○ Y   ○ N   Wedged Pillows?   ○ Y   ○ N

Last meal time? _____   Approx bedtime? _____   am   pm
(Remember to give yourself at least 2-3 hours after meals before lying down.)

End-of-day notes

Noticeable change in symptoms? _(Ex: "Throat discomfort has completely disappeared.")_

_____

_____

New terms to research   Books & websites with helpful info

_____   _____

_____   _____

Additional notes:

_____

_____

_____

Breakfast   Time: _____

List the foods you ate for breakfast.

_____   _____

_____   _____

_____   _____

Drink _____   **Drink** _____
○ room-temp ○ hot ○ cold   ○ room-temp ○ hot ○ cold

Comments:

Physical symptoms after meal: ○ **low**   ○ **intense**   ○ **non-existent**
○ Belching   ○ Upper abdominal pain and discomfort
○ Nausea   ○ Difficulty or pain with swallowing
○ Stomach fullness or bloating ○ Wheezing or dry cough

Other symptoms:

Post-breakfast energy level: ○ low   ○ medium   ○ high

Lunch   Time: _____

List the foods you ate for lunch.

_____   _____

_____   _____

_____   _____

Drink _____   **Drink** _____
○ room-temp ○ hot ○ cold   ○ room-temp ○ hot ○ cold

Comments:

Physical symptoms after meal: ○ **low**   ○ **intense**   ○ **non-existent**
○ Belching   ○ Upper abdominal pain and discomfort
○ Nausea   ○ Difficulty or pain with swallowing
○ Stomach fullness or bloating ○ Wheezing or dry cough

Other symptoms:

Post-lunch energy level: ○ low   ○ medium   ○ high

Dinner

Time: _____

List the foods you ate for dinner.

_____   _____

_____   _____

_____   _____

Drink _____   **Drink** _____
○ room-temp ○ hot ○ cold   ○ room-temp ○ hot ○ cold

Comments: _____

Physical symptoms after meal: ○ **low**   ○ **intense**   ○ **non-existent**
○ Belching   ○ Upper abdominal pain and discomfort
○ Nausea   ○ Difficulty or pain with swallowing
○ Stomach fullness or bloating   ○ Wheezing or dry cough

Other symptoms: _____

Post-dinner energy level: ○ low   ○ medium   ○ high

Snack

Time: _____

List the foods you ate as a snack.

_____   _____

Drink _____   ○ room-temp   ○ hot   ○ cold

Comments: _____

Post-snack energy level: ○ low   ○ medium   ○ high

Snack

Time: _____

List the foods you ate as a snack.

_____   _____

Drink _____   ○ room-temp   ○ hot   ○ cold

Comments: _____

Post-snack energy level: ○ low   ○ medium   ○ high

Medications & Supplements

Include prescription medication, over-the-counter medication & vitamin supplements.

_____   _____

_____   _____

_____   _____

_____   _____

_____   _____

Energy level | Restfulness

Today's waking energy level?
○ low   ○ medium   ○ high

# of times roused from sleep last night?
○ 1   ○ 2   ○ 3+

Last night's reflux/GERD symptoms:

_____   _____

_____   _____

Bed raised?   ○ Y   ○ N   Wedged Pillows?   ○ Y   ○ N

Last meal time? _____   Approx bedtime? _____ am pm
(Remember to give yourself at least 2-3 hours after meals before lying down.)

End-of-day notes

Noticeable change in symptoms? _(Ex: "Throat discomfort has completely disappeared.")_

_____

_____

New terms to research   Books & websites with helpful info

_____   _____

_____   _____

Additional notes:

_____

_____

_____

Breakfast
Time: _____

List the foods you ate for breakfast.

_____ _____

_____ _____

_____ _____

Drink _____ **Drink** _____
○ room-temp ○ hot ○ cold   ○ room-temp ○ hot ○ cold

Comments:

Physical symptoms after meal: ○ low ○ intense ○ non-existent
○ Belching   ○ Upper abdominal pain and discomfort
○ Nausea   ○ Difficulty or pain with swallowing
○ Stomach fullness or bloating ○ Wheezing or dry cough

Other symptoms:

Post-breakfast energy level: ○ low ○ medium ○ high

Lunch
Time: _____

List the foods you ate for lunch.

_____ _____

_____ _____

_____ _____

Drink _____ **Drink** _____
○ room-temp ○ hot ○ cold   ○ room-temp ○ hot ○ cold

Comments:

Physical symptoms after meal: ○ low ○ intense ○ non-existent
○ Belching   ○ Upper abdominal pain and discomfort
○ Nausea   ○ Difficulty or pain with swallowing
○ Stomach fullness or bloating ○ Wheezing or dry cough

Other symptoms:

Post-lunch energy level: ○ low ○ medium ○ high

Dinner

Time: _____

List the foods you ate for dinner.

_____   _____

_____   _____

_____   _____

Drink _____   **Drink** _____
○ room-temp ○ hot ○ cold   ○ room-temp ○ hot ○ cold

Comments: _____

Physical symptoms after meal: ○ **low** ○ **intense** ○ **non-existent**
○ Belching   ○ Upper abdominal pain and discomfort
○ Nausea   ○ Difficulty or pain with swallowing
○ Stomach fullness or bloating ○ Wheezing or dry cough

Other symptoms: _____

Post-dinner energy level: ○ low ○ medium ○ high

Snack

Time: _____

List the foods you ate as a snack.

_____   _____

Drink _____ ○ room-temp ○ hot ○ cold

Comments: _____

Post-snack energy level: ○ low ○ medium ○ high

Snack

Time: _____

List the foods you ate as a snack.

_____   _____

Drink _____ ○ room-temp ○ hot ○ cold

Comments: _____

Post-snack energy level: ○ low ○ medium ○ high

Medications & Supplements

Include prescription medication, over-the-counter medication & vitamin supplements.

_____   _____

_____   _____

_____   _____

_____   _____

_____   _____

Energy level | Restfulness

Today's waking energy level?
○ low   ○ medium   ○ high

# of times roused from sleep last night?
○ 1   ○ 2   ○ 3+

Last night's reflux/GERD symptoms:

_____   _____

_____   _____

Bed raised?   ○ Y   ○ N   Wedged Pillows?   ○ Y   ○ N

Last meal time? _____   Approx bedtime? _____ am pm
(Remember to give yourself at least 2-3 hours after meals before lying down.)

End-of-day notes

Noticeable change in symptoms? _(Ex: "Throat discomfort has completely disappeared.")_

_____

_____

New terms to research   Books & websites with helpful info

_____   _____

_____   _____

Additional notes:

_____

_____

_____

Breakfast

Time: _____

List the foods you ate for breakfast.

_____   _____

_____   _____

_____   _____

Drink _____   **Drink** _____
  ○ room-temp ○ hot ○ cold   ○ room-temp ○ hot ○ cold

Comments:

Physical symptoms after meal: ○ **low**   ○ **intense**   ○ **non-existent**
○ Belching   ○ Upper abdominal pain and discomfort
○ Nausea   ○ Difficulty or pain with swallowing
○ Stomach fullness or bloating   ○ Wheezing or dry cough

Other symptoms:

Post-breakfast energy level: ○ low   ○ medium   ○ high

Lunch

Time: _____

List the foods you ate for lunch.

_____   _____

_____   _____

_____   _____

Drink _____   **Drink** _____
  ○ room-temp ○ hot ○ cold   ○ room-temp ○ hot ○ cold

Comments:

Physical symptoms after meal: ○ **low**   ○ **intense**   ○ **non-existent**
○ Belching   ○ Upper abdominal pain and discomfort
○ Nausea   ○ Difficulty or pain with swallowing
○ Stomach fullness or bloating   ○ Wheezing or dry cough

Other symptoms:

Post-lunch energy level: ○ low   ○ medium   ○ high

Dinner

Time: _____

List the foods you ate for dinner.

_____   _____

_____   _____

_____   _____

Drink _____   **Drink** _____
○ room-temp ○ hot ○ cold   ○ room-temp ○ hot ○ cold

Comments: _____

Physical symptoms after meal: ○ **low** ○ **intense** ○ **non-existent**
○ Belching   ○ Upper abdominal pain and discomfort
○ Nausea   ○ Difficulty or pain with swallowing
○ Stomach fullness or bloating   ○ Wheezing or dry cough

Other symptoms: _____

Post-dinner energy level: ○ low ○ medium ○ high

Snack

Time: _____

List the foods you ate as a snack.

_____   _____

Drink _____   ○ room-temp ○ hot ○ cold

Comments: _____

Post-snack energy level: ○ low ○ medium ○ high

Snack

Time: _____

List the foods you ate as a snack.

_____   _____

Drink _____   ○ room-temp ○ hot ○ cold

Comments: _____

Post-snack energy level: ○ low ○ medium ○ high

Medications & Supplements

Include prescription medication, over-the-counter medication & vitamin supplements.

_____   _____

_____   _____

_____   _____

_____   _____

_____   _____

Energy level | Restfulness

Today's waking energy level?
○ low   ○ medium   ○ high

# of times roused from sleep last night?
○ 1   ○ 2   ○ 3+

Last night's reflux/GERD symptoms:

_____   _____

_____   _____

Bed raised?   ○ Y   ○ N   Wedged Pillows?   ○ Y   ○ N

Last meal time? _____   Approx bedtime? _____   am   pm
(Remember to give yourself at least 2-3 hours after meals before lying down.)

End-of-day notes

Noticeable change in symptoms? *(Ex: "Throat discomfort has completely disappeared.")*

_____

_____

New terms to research   Books & websites with helpful info

_____   _____

_____   _____

Additional notes:

_____

_____

_____

_____

Breakfast
Time: _____

List the foods you ate for breakfast.

_____   _____

_____   _____

_____   _____

Drink _____   **Drink** _____
  ○ room-temp ○ hot ○ cold   ○ room-temp ○ hot ○ cold

Comments:

Physical symptoms after meal: ○ **low**   ○ **intense**   ○ **non-existent**
○ Belching   ○ Upper abdominal pain and discomfort
○ Nausea   ○ Difficulty or pain with swallowing
○ Stomach fullness or bloating   ○ Wheezing or dry cough

Other symptoms:

Post-breakfast energy level: ○ low   ○ medium   ○ high

Lunch
Time: _____

List the foods you ate for lunch.

_____   _____

_____   _____

_____   _____

Drink _____   **Drink** _____
  ○ room-temp ○ hot ○ cold   ○ room-temp ○ hot ○ cold

Comments:

Physical symptoms after meal: ○ **low**   ○ **intense**   ○ **non-existent**
○ Belching   ○ Upper abdominal pain and discomfort
○ Nausea   ○ Difficulty or pain with swallowing
○ Stomach fullness or bloating   ○ Wheezing or dry cough

Other symptoms:

Post-lunch energy level: ○ low   ○ medium   ○ high

Dinner

Time: _____

List the foods you ate for dinner.

_____   _____

_____   _____

_____   _____

Drink _____   **Drink** _____
○ room-temp   ○ hot   ○ cold   ○ room-temp   ○ hot   ○ cold

Comments:

Physical symptoms after meal: ○ **low**   ○ **intense**   ○ **non-existent**
○ Belching   ○ Upper abdominal pain and discomfort
○ Nausea   ○ Difficulty or pain with swallowing
○ Stomach fullness or bloating   ○ Wheezing or dry cough

Other symptoms:

Post-dinner energy level: ○ low   ○ medium   ○ high

Snack

Time: _____

List the foods you ate as a snack.

_____   _____

Drink _____   ○ room-temp   ○ hot   ○ cold

Comments:

Post-snack energy level: ○ low   ○ medium   ○ high

Snack

Time: _____

List the foods you ate as a snack.

_____   _____

Drink _____   ○ room-temp   ○ hot   ○ cold

Comments:

Post-snack energy level: ○ low   ○ medium   ○ high

Medications & Supplements

Include prescription medication, over-the-counter medication & vitamin supplements.

_____   _____

_____   _____

_____   _____

_____   _____

_____   _____

Energy level | Restfulness

Today's waking energy level?
○ low ○ medium ○ high

# of times roused from sleep last night?
○ 1 ○ 2 ○ 3+

Last night's reflux/GERD symptoms:

_____   _____

_____   _____

Bed raised? ○ Y ○ N   Wedged Pillows? ○ Y ○ N

Last meal time? _____   Approx bedtime? _____ am pm
(Remember to give yourself at least 2-3 hours after meals before lying down.)

End-of-day notes

Noticeable change in symptoms? _(Ex: "Throat discomfort has completely disappeared.")_

_____

_____

New terms to research   Books & websites with helpful info

_____   _____

_____   _____

Additional notes:

_____

_____

_____

_____

Breakfast   Time: _____

List the foods you ate for breakfast.

_____   _____

_____   _____

_____   _____

Drink _____   **Drink** _____
○ room-temp ○ hot ○ cold   ○ room-temp ○ hot ○ cold

Comments: _____

Physical symptoms after meal: ○ **low** ○ **intense** ○ **non-existent**
○ Belching   ○ Upper abdominal pain and discomfort
○ Nausea   ○ Difficulty or pain with swallowing
○ Stomach fullness or bloating   ○ Wheezing or dry cough

Other symptoms: _____

Post-breakfast energy level: ○ low ○ medium ○ high

Lunch   Time: _____

List the foods you ate for lunch.

_____   _____

_____   _____

_____   _____

Drink _____   **Drink** _____
○ room-temp ○ hot ○ cold   ○ room-temp ○ hot ○ cold

Comments: _____

Physical symptoms after meal: ○ **low** ○ **intense** ○ **non-existent**
○ Belching   ○ Upper abdominal pain and discomfort
○ Nausea   ○ Difficulty or pain with swallowing
○ Stomach fullness or bloating   ○ Wheezing or dry cough

Other symptoms: _____

Post-lunch energy level: ○ low ○ medium ○ high

Dinner

Time: _____

List the foods you ate for dinner.

_____   _____

_____   _____

_____   _____

Drink _____   **Drink** _____
   ○ room-temp ○ hot ○ cold   ○ room-temp ○ hot ○ cold

Comments: _____

Physical symptoms after meal: ○ **low** ○ **intense** ○ **non-existent**
○ Belching   ○ Upper abdominal pain and discomfort
○ Nausea   ○ Difficulty or pain with swallowing
○ Stomach fullness or bloating ○ Wheezing or dry cough

Other symptoms: _____

Post-dinner energy level: ○ low ○ medium ○ high

Snack

Time: _____

List the foods you ate as a snack.

_____   _____

Drink _____   ○ room-temp ○ hot ○ cold

Comments: _____

Post-snack energy level: ○ low ○ medium ○ high

Snack

Time: _____

List the foods you ate as a snack.

_____   _____

Drink _____   ○ room-temp ○ hot ○ cold

Comments: _____

Post-snack energy level: ○ low ○ medium ○ high

Medications & Supplements

Include prescription medication, over-the-counter medication & vitamin supplements.

_____   _____

_____   _____

_____   _____

_____   _____

_____   _____

Energy level | Restfulness

Today's waking energy level?
○ low   ○ medium   ○ high

# of times roused from sleep last night?
○ 1   ○ 2   ○ 3+

Last night's reflux/GERD symptoms:

_____   _____

_____   _____

Bed raised?   ○ Y   ○ N   Wedged Pillows?   ○ Y   ○ N

Last meal time? _____   Approx bedtime? _____ am pm
(Remember to give yourself at least 2-3 hours after meals before lying down.)

End-of-day notes

Noticeable change in symptoms? _(Ex: "Throat discomfort has completely disappeared.")_

_____

_____

New terms to research   Books & websites with helpful info

_____   _____

_____   _____

Additional notes:

_____

_____

_____

CPSIA information can be obtained
at www.ICGtesting.com
Printed in the USA
LVOW09s1631030817

543714LV00007B/425/P